Yeasts in Biotechnology

Edited by Thalita Peixoto Basso

Published in London, United Kingdom

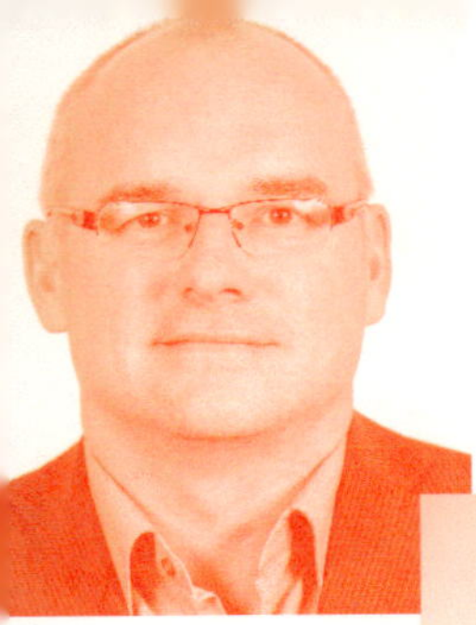

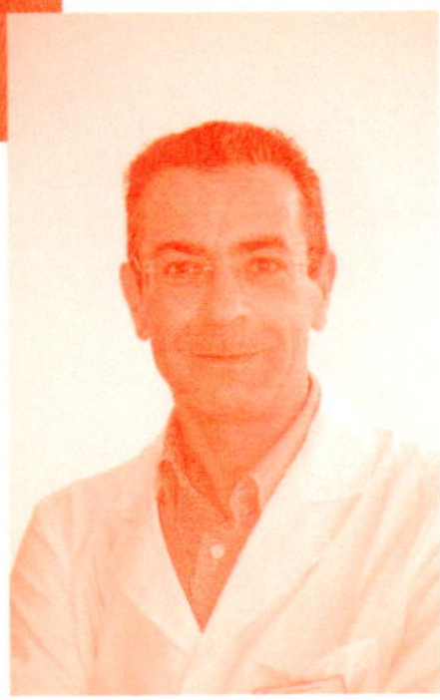

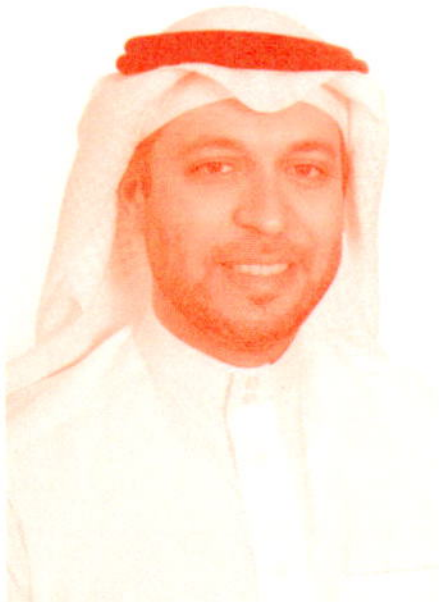

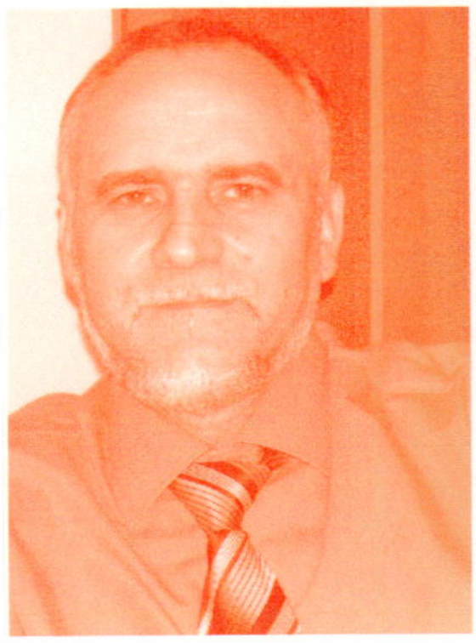

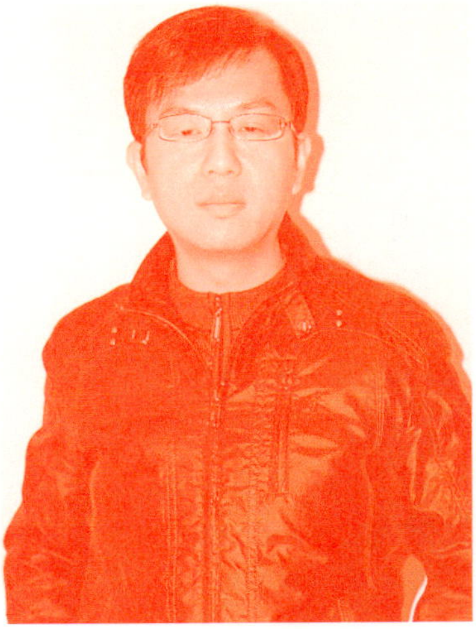

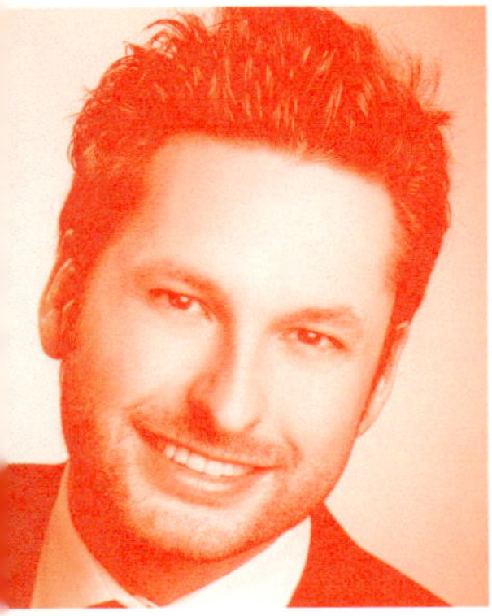

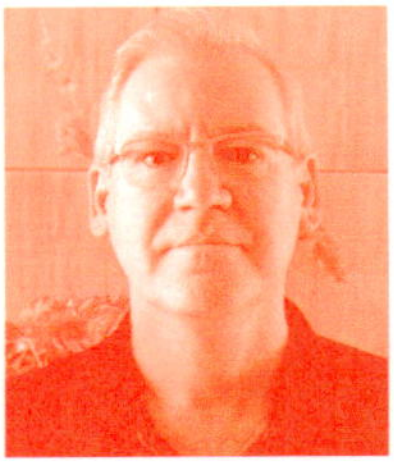

IntechOpen

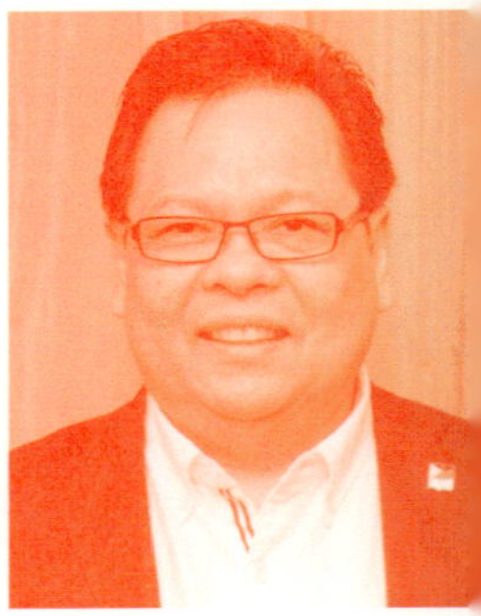

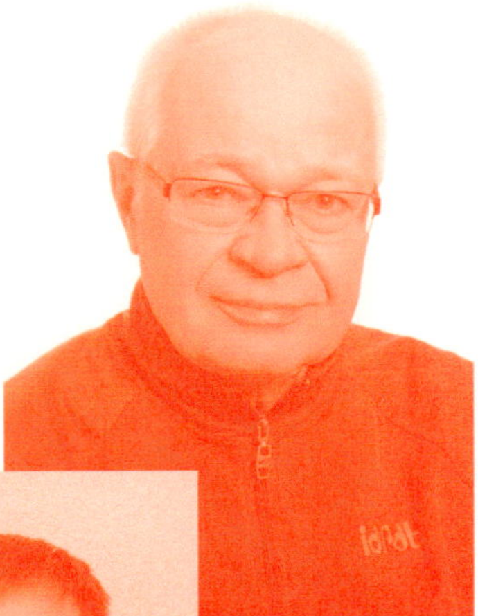

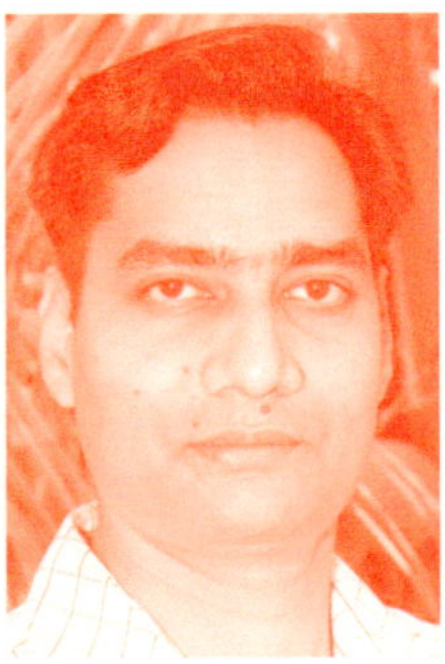

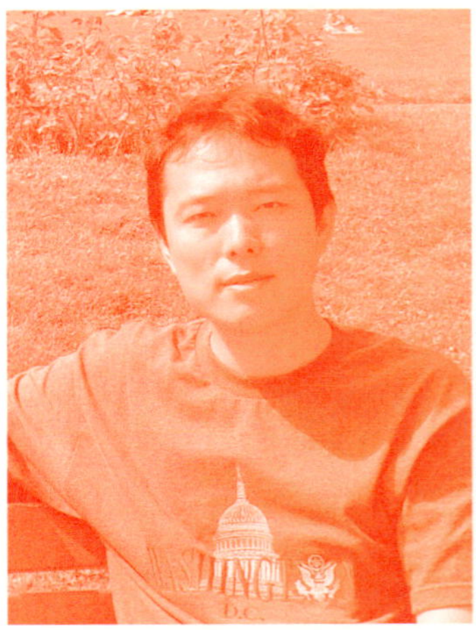

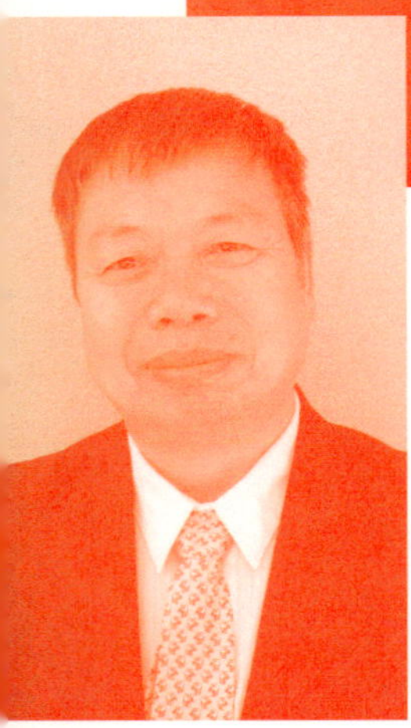

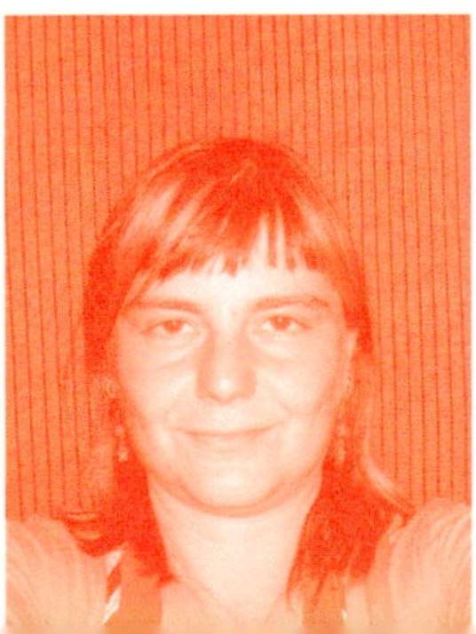

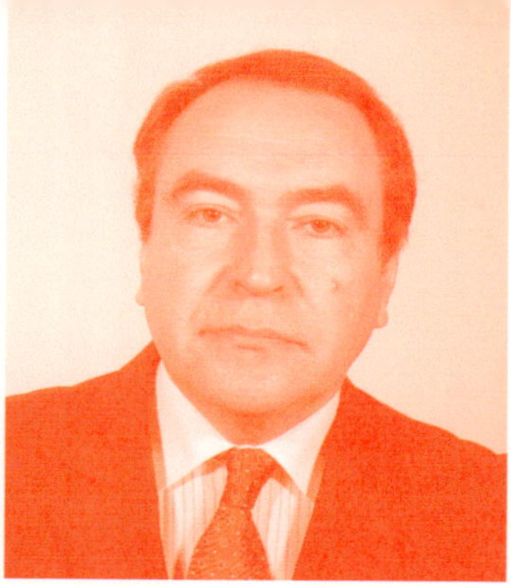
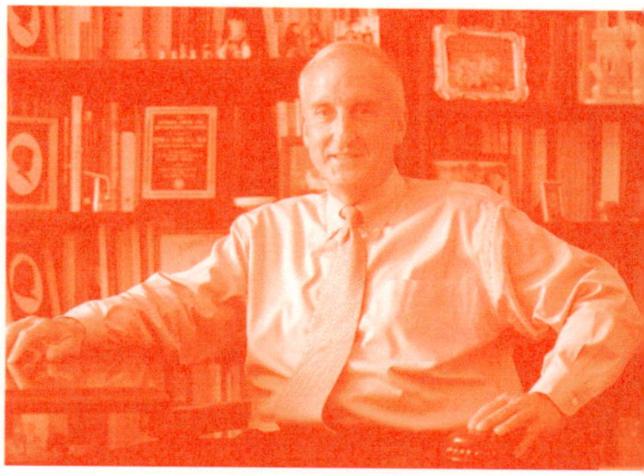
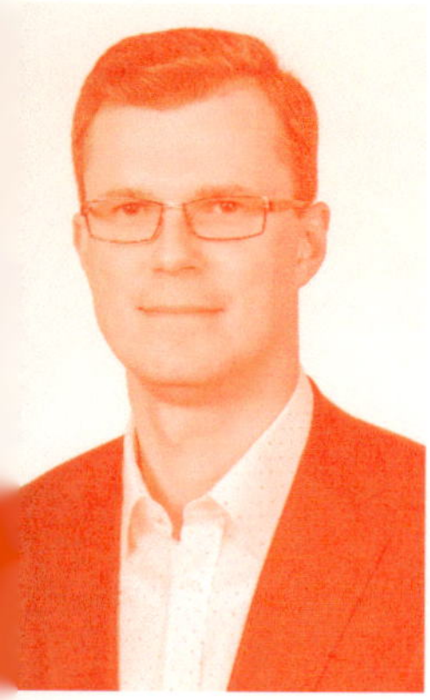
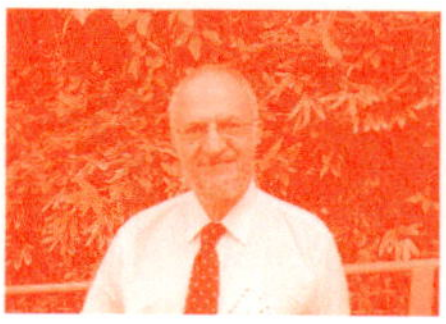
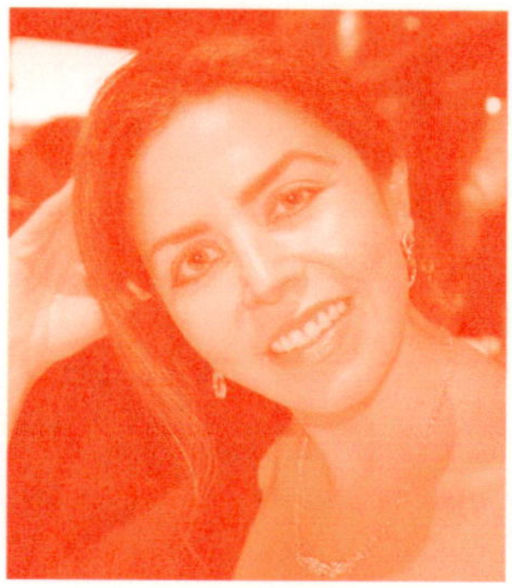

Supporting open minds since 2005

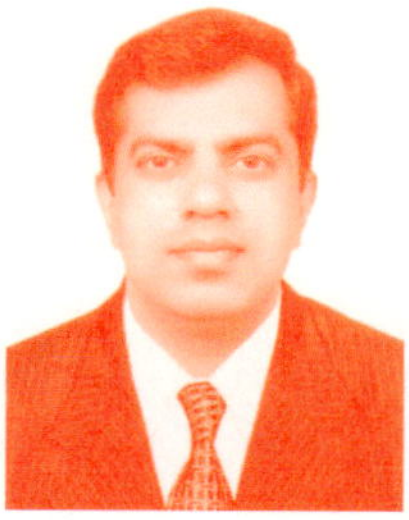
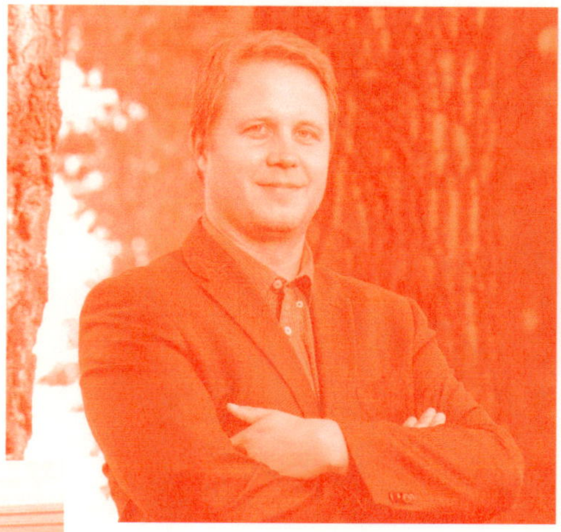
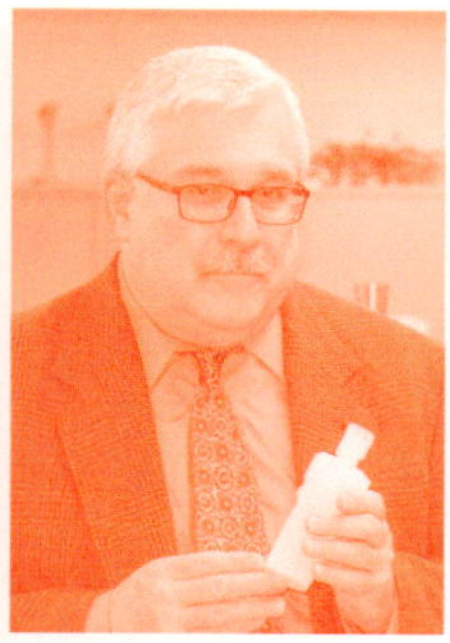
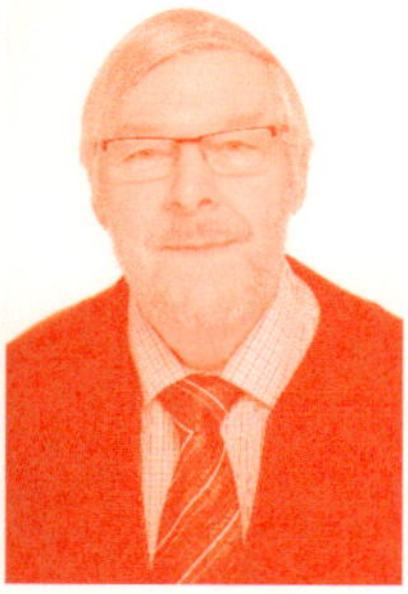
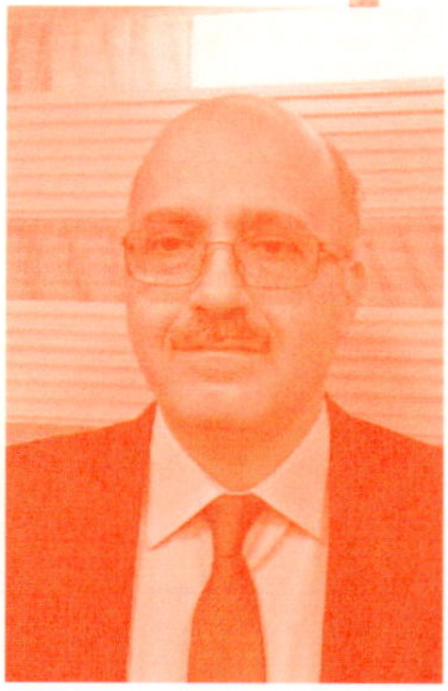
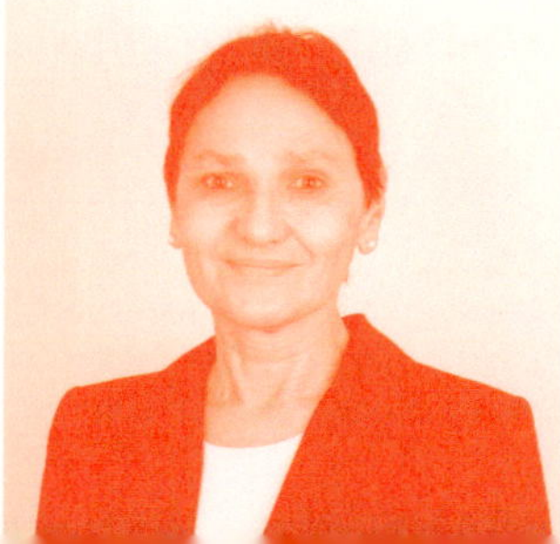
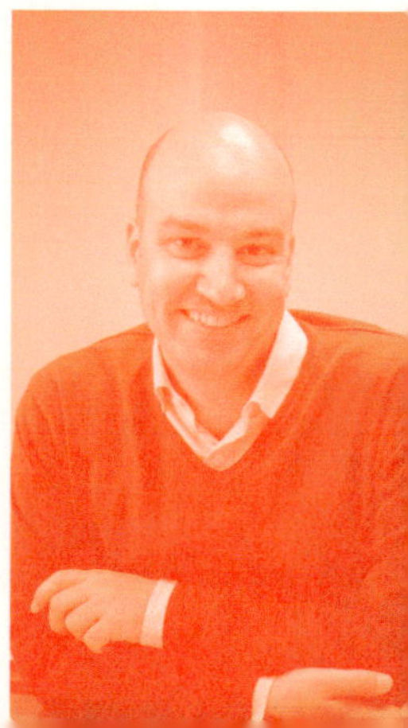

Yeasts in Biotechnology
http://dx.doi.org/10.5772/intechopen.77938
Edited by Thalita Peixoto Basso

Contributors
Oscar Ruiz Barrera, Yamicela Castillo Castillo, Jaime Salinas-Chavira, Shakira Ghazanfar, Ghulam Muhammad Ali, Irum Arif, Sidra Irshad, Khanzadi Nazneen Manzoor, Aayesha Riaz, Naeem Riaz, Saima Naveed, Camila de Souza Varize, Renata Maria Christofoleti-Furlan, Elisangela de Souza Miranda Muynarsk, Gilberto Vinícius de Melo Pereira, Lucas Dantas Lopes, Luiz Carlos Basso, Chun Li, Wentao Sun, Yu-jia Zhao, Raúl Ferrer-Gallego, Imma Andorrà, Gemma Miró, Noelia Espligares, Ana Maria Mislata, Miquel Puxeu, Mathew Lyman, Salustra Urbin, Cheryl Strout, Bonnee Rubinfeld, Thalita Peixoto Basso, Carlos Alberto Labate

Notice
Statements and opinions expressed in the chapters are these of the individual contributors and not necessarily those of the editors or publisher. No responsibility is accepted for the accuracy of information contained in the published chapters. The publisher assumes no responsibility for any damage or injury to persons or property arising out of the use of any materials, instructions, methods or ideas contained in the book.

First published in London, United Kingdom, 2019 by IntechOpen
IntechOpen is the global imprint of INTECHOPEN LIMITED, registered in England and Wales, registration number: 11086078, The Shard, 25th floor, 32 London Bridge Street
London, SE19SG – United Kingdom
Printed in Croatia

British Library Cataloguing-in-Publication Data
A catalogue record for this book is available from the British Library

Additional hard and PDF copies can be obtained from orders@intechopen.com

Yeasts in Biotechnology
Edited by Thalita Peixoto Basso
p. cm.
Print ISBN 978-1-78923-927-0
Online ISBN 978-1-78923-928-7
eBook (PDF) ISBN 978-1-83881-228-7

For EU product safety concerns:
IN TECH d.o.o., Prolaz Marije Krucifikse Kozulić 3, 51000 Rijeka, Croatia, info@intechopen.com or visit our website at intechopen.com.

Meet the editor

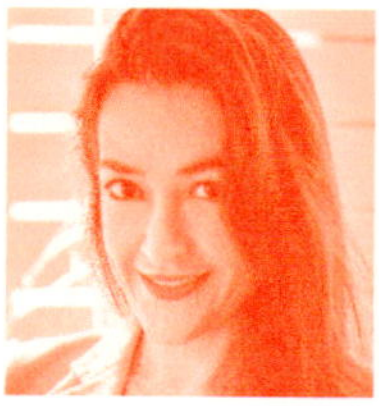

Thalita Peixoto Basso received her Bachelor's degree in Agriculture Engineering (2008) from Londrina State University (PR-Brazil). During this period, she studied fermentation characteristics of *Saccharomyces cerevisiae* isolated from ethanol industrial processes. She obtained her Master's degree in Science from the Agri-food Industry, Food and Nutrition Department of the University of Sao Paulo (ESALQ/USP, SP-Brazil) in 2010. During this time, she isolated and selected fungi with high cellulose activity for the enzymatic hydrolysis of sugarcane bagasse.
She received her PhD in Science from the Soil Science Department (Agricultural Microbiology Program) at ESALQ/USP (2015), with a period of one year as a visiting scholar at the University of California Berkeley and Energy Bioscience Institute. Meanwhile, she worked on the improvement of *S. cerevisiae* by hybridization for increased tolerance toward inhibitors from second-generation ethanol substrates. Currently, she is a postdoctoral working with metabolomics and proteomics of fermentation processes in the Genetics Department at ESALQ/USP.

Contents

Preface

Yeasts are one of the most important eukaryotic microorganisms due to their role as model organisms for eukaryotic biological studies with a focus on understanding and interpreting human DNA. Recently, researches have been working with several yeast genera and species such as *Saccharomyces cerevisiae*, *Pichia pastoris*, and *Schizosaccharomyces pombe* as model organisms for cancer biology investigation, including tumorigenic mechanism studies, development, and production of anticancer drugs.

Many thousands of years ago, Egyptian, Babylonian, and Greek civilizations used these microorganisms to produce fermented foods and beverages, such as bread, beer, and wine. Since then, yeasts have been applied to the food industry and their utilization has been increasing over the last few decades. On the other hand, new yeast platforms such as cell factories have been developed for the production of biochemicals such as fuels and drugs.

This book offers a broad understanding of yeast applications such as cell factories for the production of biofuel, food, and bioproducts with high value. Additionally, the book provides an overview of yeast utilization as probiotics in animal nutrition. The book starts with an introduction chapter on the advances of yeast utilization in human history up to current biotechnology approaches.

The six chapters are grouped into three sections: Animal Nutrition, Food Industry, and Industrial Bioproducts. The Animal Nutrition section comprises two chapters dealing with the application of yeast as a probiotic in animal nutrition. In these chapters, the reader is guided through the action mechanisms of indigenous and commercial *S. cerevisiae* yeasts on ruminant gut microbial balance and can identify the ideal probiotic yeast for animal feeding.

In the Food Industry section, the advantages of nonconventional yeast strains on the food and beverage industry such as wine making, brewing, coffee and cocoa fermentation, and xylitol production are presented. It also covers the biotransformation process and analytical procedures, such as mechanisms of accumulation, extraction, and quantification of organically bound selenium by *S. cerevisiae.*

The Industrial Bioproducts section deals with the application of yeast as a platform for the biosynthesis of biochemicals such as flavonoids, alkaloids, terpenoids, and saponins used in the agriculture industry. It also covers the application of *Rhodotorula/Rhodosporidium* as a platform cell factory for biofuel feedstock, carotenoids, enzymes, and biosurfactant production.

This book intends to present a broad understanding of several biotechnology applications of yeasts in industrial bioprocesses. It will cover a multitude of issues such as the development of a platform cell factory, the use of nonconventional yeasts, and the diverse application of yeasts on bioprocesses. Other aspects related to bioprocesses will also be analyzed, such as biofuels and bioproduct production and yeast application in wine making and brewing.

Thalita Peixoto Basso, Ph.D.
University of Sao Paulo,
Brazil

Section 1

Introduction

Chapter 1

Introductory Chapter: Yeasts in Biotechnology

Thalita Peixoto Basso, Luiz Carlos Basso and Carlos Alberto Labate

1. Introduction

Yeasts are very important for many reasons. These microorganisms were the first species to be domesticated by man, although not intentionally. For millennia they were used in fermented beverages and foods without knowing their existence. Biochemistry as a science was born when physiologists looked deeper in sugar fermentation in the final of nineteenth century.

Today yeast takes a place in several fields of science and technology. As long as yeast genes and mammal cells encode very similar proteins, these microorganisms are useful as a model to understand and interpret human DNA sequences. Indeed, yeast genetic manipulation is much easier and cheaper than mammalian systems. So yeast has turned out to be a useful model for eukaryotic biology [1, 2].

Furthermore yeasts such as *Saccharomyces cerevisiae*, *Picchia pastoris*, and *Schizosaccharomyces pombe* have been used as model organisms to study cancer biology, including research and development of tumorigenic mechanisms and production of anticancer drugs [3].

Particularly, *Saccharomyces cerevisiae* is a model organism to study epigenetic traits that can be characterized as a stably heritable phenotype resulting from changes in a chromosome without alteration in the DNA sequence. As a result of yeast small eukaryotic genome, short generation time and easy genetic manipulation [4].

Additionally yeasts are very important players in many economical relevant bioprocessing as bakery, brewery, distilling, food industry, and biofuel, leading yeasts to be considered the most explored and studied eukaryotic microorganism.

2. Yeast application

Since 8000 years ago in our history, humans have been using microorganisms to produce fermented foods and beverages. More recently chemicals and fuels have been produced by bioprocesses. The development of cell factories has been incentivized for the industrial production of new chemicals. However the development of new yeast platform cell factory is costly and time-consuming. The difficulty to develop new cell factories to produce a specific metabolite is due to metabolism which has evolved to allow cell growth and maintenance to keep homeostasis [5].

Yeasts from phyla of ascomycetes and basidiomycetes have diverse biotechnological application on food industry. They are responsible for a wide range of fermented products such as alcoholic beverages (e.g., beer, wine, and "cachaça"), fermented milk, cheese, bread, and so on. Yeast also has an application in the functional food industry as probiotics and nutraceutical products [6].

 IntechOpen

Saccharomyces cerevisiae has been metabolically engineered for the production of first-generation and second-generation bioethanols, advanced biofuels, and chemicals [7–11].

Recently, new tools for genome editing as CRISPR-Cas9 technology have the advantage to allow introduction of many genes into any chromosome location [12, 13]. On the other hand, high-throughput methods as transcriptomic, proteomic, and metabolomic analyses support the introduction of metabolic pathway over cellular physiology metabolism. Indeed next-generation sequencing allows the identification of any genome modification responsible for desirable phenotype [5].

3. Conclusion

In conclusion, we believe that the yeasts are a nearly ideal model system for eukaryotic biology at the cellular and molecular level. Additionally their use in increasingly technological applications will augment the importance of yeast for human well-being.

Acknowledgements

The authors would like to acknowledge CAPES and Inter-unit Bioenergy Post Graduation Program (USP/UNESP/UNICAMP) for PNPD/CAPES postdoctoral fellowship (process number 88882.317582/2019-01), Max Feffer Laboratory from Genetic Department (ESALQ/USP), and Yeast Physiology and Fermentation Laboratory from Biological Science (ESALQ/USP).

Conflict of interest

The authors confirm there is no conflict of interest.

Author details

Thalita Peixoto Basso*, Luiz Carlos Basso and Carlos Alberto Labate
"Luiz de Queiroz" College of Agriculture, University of Sao Paulo, Piracicaba, SP, Brazil

*Address all correspondence to: tpbasso@usp.br

References

[1] Botstein D, Fink GR. Yeast: An experimental organism for modern biology. Science. 1988;**240**:1439-1443. DOI: 10.1126/science.3287619

[2] Botstein D, Chervitz SA, Cherry JM. Yeast as a model organism. Science. 1997;**277**:1259-1260. DOI: 10.1116/science.277.5330.1259

[3] Ferreira R, Limeta A, Nielsen J. Tackling cancer with yeast-based technologies. Trends in Biotechnology. 2018;**1735**:1-12. DOI: 10.1016/j.tibtech.2018.11.013

[4] Fuchs SM, Quasem I. Budding yeast as a model study epigenetics. Drug Discovery Today: Disease Models. 2014;**12**:1-16. DOI: 10.1016/j.ddmod.2014.04.004

[5] Nielsen J, Keasling JD. Engineering cellular metabolism. Cell. 2016;**164**:1185-1197. DOI: 10.1016/j.cell.2016.02.004

[6] Rai AK, Pandey A, Sahoo D. Biotechnological potential of yeasts in functional food industry. Trends in Food Science and Technology. 2019;**83**:129-137. DOI: 10.1016/j.tifs.2018.11.016

[7] Zhou H, Cheng JS, Wang BL, Fink GR, Stephanopoulos G. Xylose isomerase overexpression along with engineering of the pentose phosphate pathway and evolutionary engineering enable rapid xylose utilization and ethanol production by *Saccharomyces cerevisiae*. Metabolic Engineering. 2012;**14**:611-622. DOI: 10.1016/j.ymben.2012.07.011

[8] Nielsen J, Larsson C, van Maris A, Pronk J. Metabolic engineering of yeast for production of fuels and chemicals. Current Opinion in Biotechnology. 2013;**24**:398-404. DOI: 10.1016/j.copbio.2013.03.023

[9] Basso TP. Improvement of *Saccharomyces cerevisiae* by hybridization for increased tolerance towards inhibitors from second-generation ethanol substrate [thesis]. Piracicaba-SP: University of Sao Paulo; 2015

[10] Jin YS, Cate JHD. Metabolic engineering of yeast for lignocellulosic biofuel production. Current Opinion in Chemical Biology. 2017;**41**:99-106. DOI: 10.1016/j.cbpa.2017.10.025

[11] Kim SR, Skerker JM, Kong II, Kim H, Maurer MJ, Zhang GC, et al. Metabolic engineering of a haploid strain derived from a triploid industrial yeast for producing cellulosic ethanol. Metabolic Engineering. 2017;**40**:176-185. DOI: 10.1016/j.ymben.2017.02.006

[12] Estrela R, Cate JHD. Energy biotechnology in the CRISPR-Cas9 era. Current Opinion in Biotechnology. 2016;**38**:79-84. DOI: 10.1016/j.copbio.2016.01.005

[13] Jakociunas T, Jensen MK, Keasling JD. CRISPR/Cas9 adbances engineering of microbial cell factories. Metabolic Engineering. 2016;**34**:44-59. DOI: 10.1016/j.ymben.2015.12.003

Section 2

Animal Nutrition

Chapter 2

Common Methods to Understand and Develop Indigenous Probiotics Yeast for Ruminant

Shakira Ghazanfar, Aayesha Riaz, Ghulam Muhammad Ali, Saima Naveed, Irum Arif, Sidra Irshad, Naeem Riaz and Khanzadi Nazneen Manzoor

Abstract

Probiotic yeast enhanced the ruminal gut microbial balance by producing intercellular effectors and important metabolites. The impact of yeast addition on animal health is influenced by different interlinked factors including animal genomics, its gut microbiota, and environment. Therefore, all factors should be considered regarding achieving the maximum outputs from animal probiotic yeast. In the situation of a high feeding cost, microbial feed supplements provide a suitable nutritional approach, which allows increased nutrient digestion rate and accordingly improves animal performance. Many yeast products are commercially available, but their efficiency as probiotic dietary addition in a particular breed is mostly questionable. Therefore, identification of ideal probiotic yeast strain is of great interest in this context. Innovative methods in relation to develop new probiotic are mainly focused on the exploring novel microbial strains from indigenous sources. It has been noted that for the identification of best probiotic strain for the host, a linkage between culture-independent and culture-dependent methods is a functional step. In this chapter, we will discuss the mode of action of probiotic yeast on animal lower gut microbiota and identification of ideal probiotic yeast by using advanced molecular methods.

Keywords: indigenous probiotic yeast, lower gut, microbiota, molecular methods

1. Introduction

Over the past decades, the livestock industry has been revolutionized toward the use of microbial feed additives due to an increasing awareness of the stockholders on the beneficial role of probiotics in production and gut health status [1, 2]. There are several probiotic products that are commercially available and marketed for animal use [3]. Most probiotic products at the moment do not go through pre-market approvals and are commonly used for a much wider range of scenarios in which their efficacy is not well established. Similarly, latest molecular methods such as gene sequencing and phylogenetic analysis are not used to identify the probiotic strains as feed supplements. For the selection of best probiotic product, it is highly important to determine the real probiotic potential of the microbial strain by using latest molecular methods. In this contract, locally isolated and validated probiotic strains will be better than any unauthorized local available strain. The competitive advantage and adaptability to local microbial ecosystem will allow local probiotic strain to grow and adhere well in the local animal breed. Literature showed that probiotic strains should specifically prepare according to purpose and function related to the milk enhancement in local breed [4, 5]. Nowadays, it is highly accepted that probiotic yeast is highly productive in terms of milk and meat for large animals [6, 7]. Probiotic yeast improves the ruminal gut microbiota which may increase the nutrient digestibility and leads to improve animal productivity [8]. In large animals, ingested feed digested by numerous microbial species is present along the gastrointestinal tract [9]. This microbial community consists of 1014 members, mainly composed of fibrolytic bacterial species [10]. Literature highlighted that gut microbiota plays important role in the feed digestion and utilization. The gut microbial populations in cow have been identified in almost 90% of the total microbial community [11]. On the other hand, a certain fraction of the GI tract bacterial community has yet to be identified due to less knowledge of the microbial community in gut microbial ecosystem because majority of the 16S rRNA gene sequences from feces are taken from unidentified species, and many modern methods of genomic analysis of communities to determine changes in microbiota have been used by many scientists [12]. Studies have utilized culture-independent sequencing techniques, 16S rDNA bacterial tag-encoded FLX amplicon pyrosequencing and many more have added a new era to determine the microbial diversity of the GI tract [13]. Research noted that the culture-independent methods deliver a comprehensive assessment of the microbial community composition, while the culture-dependent methods provide the structural and functional diversity of the microbial strains [14]. In this chapter, a detailed discussion on the effects of probiotic yeast in ruminant's well being, production performance, uses of different omics methodologies for the discovery of ideal animal probiotic strains and development of indigenous probiotic yeast for ruminant will be employed.

2. Yeast: an ideal microbial feed supplement for ruminants

The *Saccharomyces cerevisiae* (baker's yeast) is the first eukaryotic sequenced genome. The sequencing of first whole eukaryotic genome was a challenging task for the scientists, but the efforts of more than 600 scientists from Europe, North America, and Japan made it possible. The entire sequence of the yeast was released in 1996. The size of the baker's yeast genome is 12.1 Mb containing 16 chromosomes and 5400 coding genes approximately. The sequence information of yeast is available at *Saccharomyces* Genome Database (SGD), Yeast Protein Database (YPD), and Munich Information Center for Protein Sequences (MIPS) [15] (**Table 1**).

Ruminant nutritionists have been pondering to improvise new methodologies for ameliorating the roles of microflora in ruminants and enhance processes of

Yeast genome	
Genome size	12.1 Mb
Chromosomes	16
Genes	5300–5400
Base pairs	12 million base pairs
Databases	SGD, MIPS, YPD

Table 1.
Details of first eukaryotic sequenced genome (yeast).

digestion and fermentation along with augmented nutrients usage and bioavailability using feed supplementation. One of the commonly used methods was the use of growth promoters (antibiotics) to restrict the pathogenic effect on productivity of ruminants [16]. Nevertheless, antibiotics have been reported to cause serious health challenges to consumers and environmental implications. Thus, their usage has been banned in 2006 due to emerging antibiotic resistance. In the light of these concerns, consumer preferred more natural product. A super alternate of feed additives was the use of probiotics [17]. Probiotics are living microorganisms confined in animal feed that affect the host by improving the digestion [18]. Other definition includes probiotics as microorganisms (viable) that functions in gaining weight and feed conversions along with reducing diarrheal incidence [19]. Probiotics have been deployed as one of the recent exploited proposals in ensuring efficiency of production systems and safety to both consumers and environment [20, 21]. In ruminant nutrition, yeast probiotics are commonly being used because of their efficient roles in rumen stabilization and maintaining microbial communities specifically fibrolytic bacteria [22]. The yeast cells function in maintaining throughout viability of the digestive tract [23]. Yeast supplementation as probiotics enhanced feed conversion, efficient fermentation, and fiber digestion in the rumen, maintained ruminal pH, increased milk production [24, 25] and feed intake and production of organic acids and vitamins to activate the growth of the lactic acid bacteria (LAB) [26]. The commonly used yeast probiotic is *Saccharomyces cerevisiae*. Numerous literatures on *Saccharomyces cerevisiae* as supplement are available that dated back to the 1950s and continued under study till today [27]. Significant role of yeast supplementation (live) in diet has been stated for lactating and growing ruminants. Recent studies confirmed that they increase the ruminant's milk production early lactation period by altering the fermentation of food inside the GIT of ruminants[28]. Latest beef and dairy production systems demand active muscle growth and high milk yield via feeding animal at high ruminal ferment ability rates. This would result in increased risk of metabolic disorders such as acidosis due to dysbiosis in ruminal microbial environment resulting in abnormal functioning in rumen which further leads to poor feed intake, health, and decreased productivity [29]. Therefore, yeast supplementation in ruminant diet is beneficial in the ruminal functioning and overall animal health and maintenance. The ameliorating functions of yeast probiotic on digestibility of high forage diets also underscore the potential use of yeast supplementation to optimize the use of lower quality feeds.

3. Understanding of the ruminant microbial community for development of ideal probiotic yeast for ruminants

Rumen microbial manipulation by using the probiotics to improve the ruminant feed digestion is a promising production improvement strategy. A better understanding of the rumen microbiology is an important step to select and prepare a new yeast strain affecting on functional specific microbes. Latest molecular techniques have provided the opportunity to study the rumen microbiota in detail for development of the ideal probiotic.

3.1 Digestive system of ruminants

Digestive system of ruminant is composed of four parts: reticulum, rumen, omasum and abomasums. The rumen is that part of the digestive system in which fermentation is carried out [30]. The rumen can also be defined as a complex ecosystem in which nutrients consumed by different microorganisms are digested anaerobically. Microbial biomass and volatile fatty acids are most common end products of fermentation which are then used by ruminant host. Interaction of host animal and microorganisms is a symbiotic relationship that helps the ruminant hosts in digestion of fiber-rich and protein-low diets. Rumen microorganisms provide enzymes that are necessary for fermentation processes, which in turn allow ruminants to obtain energy contained in forage [31]. Growth and activity of ruminal microorganisms are influenced by different factors including pH, temperature, osmotic pressure, buffering capacity, and redox potential. These factors are determined by environmental factors. Temperature of the rumen is in the range of 39–39.5°C. But when animal eats, fermentation occurs that generates heat due to which temperature increases up to the limit of 41°C [32, 33]. Short-chain fatty acid generation along with their absorption, saliva production, feed intake level and type, as well as exchange of phosphates and bicarbonates through epithelium of the rumen are the factors that affect pH [34]. In the reticule ruminal environment, these factors determine the buffering capacity as well as pH. There is a constant change in pH but mostly it remains in the range of 5.5–7.0 [35]. When there is an acidic environment in the cell, bacterial intracellular pH decreases. Microbial enzymes are very much sensitive to pH, i.e., bacterial growth is inhibited when there is an acidic pH. This is due to the disproportion of intracellular hydrogen ions [36]. In the rumen, ions and molecules affect osmotic pressure due to which gas tension is created. Fermentation process in the rumen depends upon the environmental factors and the diet due to which these factors also affect rumen osmotic pressure [37] (**Figure 1**).

3.2 Microbial community of GIT

Bacteria are more in number than any other microbes. It is noted that there are five groups of rumen bacteria: (1) free-living in liquid phase, (2) loosely attached with feed, (3) firmly attached with feed, (4) attached with rumen epithelial lining, and (5) attached with protozoa/fungi. The bacterial species inside the rumen are 99.5% obligatory anaerobic. Mostly rumen bacteria are involved in the fermentation of fibers, starch, and sugar present in the feed and converted into volatile fatty acid, H_2, and CO_2 [38]. Most of the bacteria are responsible for degradation of different types of dietary components [39] (**Table 2**).

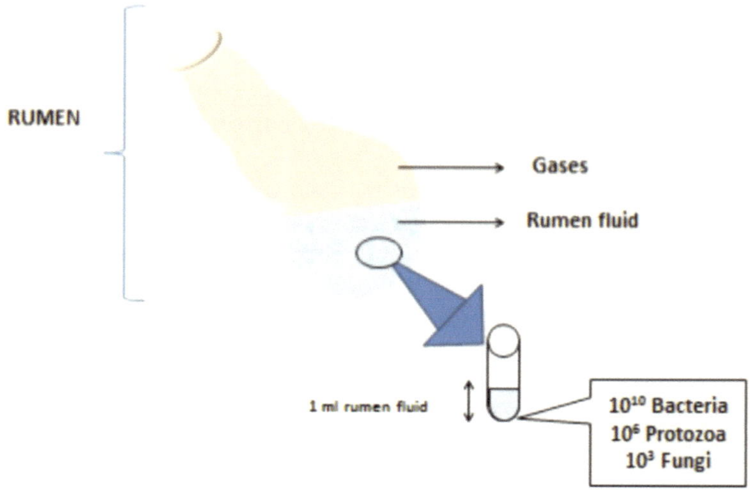

Figure 1.
Rumen ecosystem: different types of microbial flora present inside the rumen. The most abundant microbes are bacteria.

Majority of anaerobic rumen fungi is from order *Neocallimastigales* within the *phylum Neocallimastigomycota*. On the phylogeny basis, six genera have been identified, which are *Piromyces*, *Neocallimastix*, *Caecomyces*, *Anaeromyces*, *Orpinomyces*, *and Cyllamyces* [40]. In fiber digestion, fungi play a very important role because of the vegetative thallic rhizoids. The main functions of the rumen fungi are the lignin and fiber degradation by producing different types of enzymes [41] (**Table 3**).

3.3 Mechanism of action of probiotic yeast in the rumen

The rumen is the first part of the ruminant stomach which has a well-developed microbial ecosystem containing different types of microbes (bacteria, fungi, protozoa, and bacteriophages). These microbes coexist in ecological equilibrium

Bacteria	Species
Carbohydrate-utilizing bacteria	*Fibrobacter succinogenes* *Ruminococcus flavefaciens* *Ruminococcus albus* *Clostridium cellobioparum* *Clostridium longisporum* *Clostridium lochheadii* *Eubacterium cellulosolvens* *Cillobacterium cellulosolvens* *Butyrivibrio fibrisolvens* *Prevotella ruminicola* *Bacteroides ruminicola* *Eubacterium xylanophilum* *Bacteroides uniformis*
Nitrogen-utilizing bacteria	*Prevotella ruminicola* *Ruminobacteramylophilus* *Clostridium bifermentans*
Lipid-utilizing bacteria	*Anaerovibriolipolytica*

Table 2.
Bacterial diversity of the rumen microbial ecosystem.

Microbial species	Rumen	Fecal
Bacteria	*Bulleidia* *Roseburia* *Prevotella* *Ruminococcus* *Acidaminococcus* *Megasphaera* *Succiniclasticum*	*Bacteroides* *Bifidobacterium* *Clostridium* *Collinsella* *Blautia* *Dorea* *Lactobacillus* *Peptostreptococcus* *Treponema* *Succinivibrio* *Faecalibacterium*
Fungi	*Caecomyces* *Orpinomyces* *Piromyces*	*Caecomyces* *Orpinomyces* *Piromyces*
Archaea	*Methanobrevibacter* *Methanosphaera*	*Methanobrevibacter* *Methanosphaera*

Table 3.
Bacteria, fungi, and archaea present inside the rumen and feces of dairy cows.

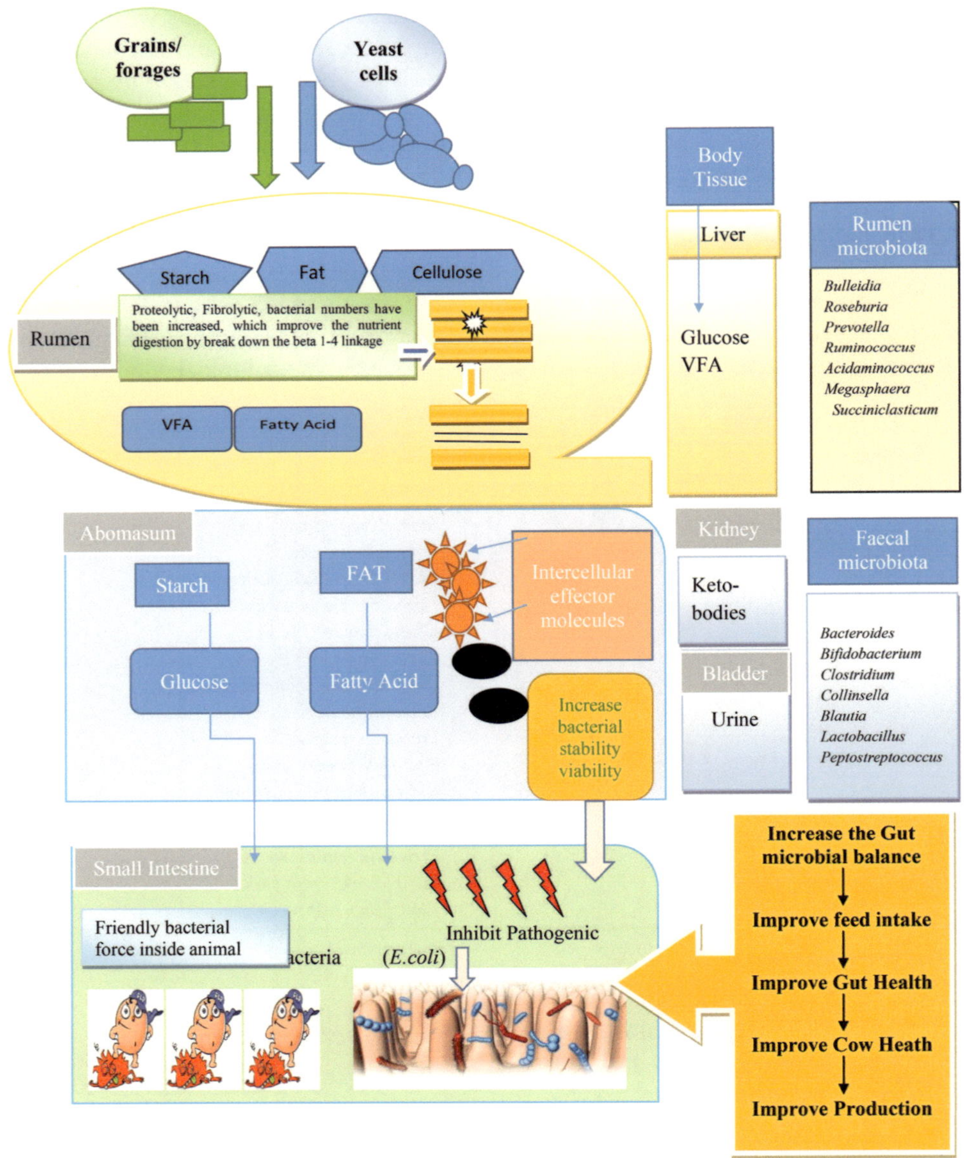

Figure 2.
Representative scheme of effect of live yeast on the microbial flora of the gastrointestinal tract in ruminants: live yeast improves carbohydrate, protein, and lipid digestion rates by improving the production of cellulolytic, hemi-cellulolytic, and proteolytic and lipolytic bacteria and fungi.

in unique symbiotic relationship between cows and rumen microbes. The cows supply food to the rumen microbes which in turn digest the feedstuff to provide cows the essential nutrients in the form of microbial protein as organic acid energy sources. The microscopic view of rumen ecosystem showed that it is consisted of a number of bacteria, protozoa and fungi [42]. Bacteria make the largest population in this diverse microbial world. Their function is to digest the fibers, starch, sugar acids, and protein to give useful compounds and elements necessary for the growth and productivity of the cows. The role of protozoa and fungi is less clear. However, these microbes do provide help in digestion of feed. The structure and function of microbial community are influenced by feed composition

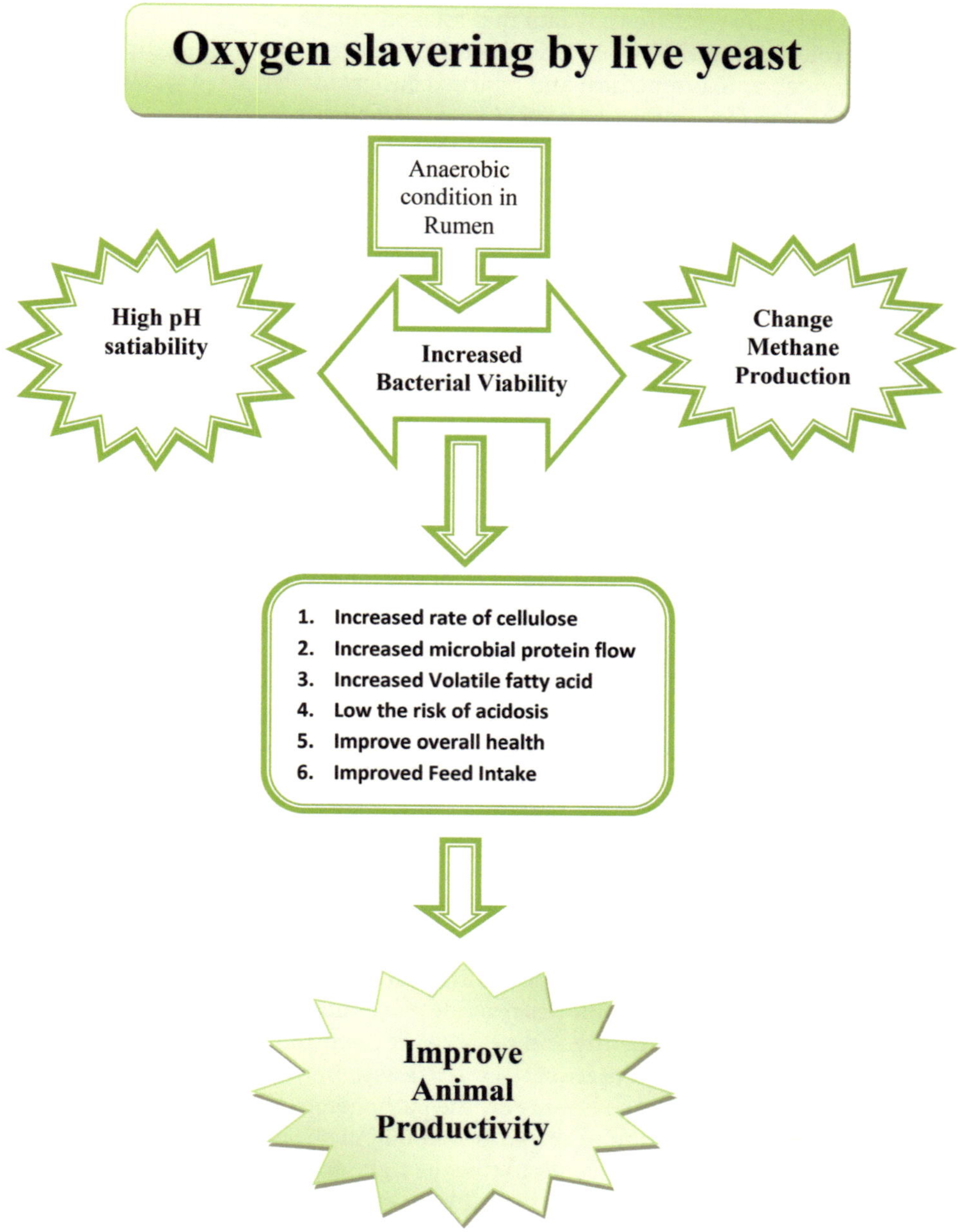

Figure 3.
A scheme describing the mode of action of yeast culture: improved the gut microbial balance is related to the O_2 slavering by live yeast cells.

and mainly by the host genetic potential. *Prevotella* and *Succinivibrionaceae* are the dominated rumen bacterial communities, cellulolytic and fibrolytic genera; *Neocallimastigaceae* are the dominant fecal and rumen fungal communities; and *Methanobrevibacter* are the dominant fecal and rumen archaeal communities in the adult ruminants. *Bacteroidetes* and *Firmicutes* are the dominant phyla of bacterial communities. *Bacteroidaceae*, *Lachnospiraceae*, *Prevotellaceae*, *Ruminococcaceae*, *Succinivibrionaceae*, and *Veillonellaceae* are the most abundant bacterial families in adult ruminant [43]. The term "yeast" is originally derived from the Dutch word *gist*, which basically refers to the foam that formed during beer fermentation. A variety of roles is played by yeast in veterinary practices, livestock feeding, and medicine as well as in biomedical and pharmaceutical industries [44]. Hayduck first discovered the inhibitory activity of yeast. Probiotics such as yeast or fungi have been extensively used in ruminant feed for the improvement of growth, health, and lactation due to their impact on rumen pH, intake of dry matter, and digestibility of nutrients [45]. Probiotic yeast has potential beneficial effects on the rumen. In the cattle, the ability of live yeast for enhancement of milk yield as well as weight gain is due to the fact that yeast is responsible for stimulating bacterial activity in the rumen [46]. Mechanism of action of yeast mainly stimulates the growth of cellulatic and hemicellulatic bacteria [47]. Increase in the number of bacteria in the rumen is due to the reproducible effects of probiotic yeast. Yeasts remove oxygen from the rumen due to which bacterial performance improves in the rumen. To maintain the metabolic activity, yeast cells consume available oxygen on the surface of freshly ingested feed in the rumen. Few studies showed that there is a significant decrease in redox potential, up to -20 mV by providing yeast supplementation (**Figure 2**).

Better conditions have been created by this change for the growth of anaerobic cellulolytic bacteria which in turn stimulates their attachment to forage particles as well as increases the initial rate of cellulolysis. Recalcitrant plant lignocellulosic material is not degraded by ruminants on its own. They rely on rumen microbial flora for its degradation [48]. The main components of the fiber are cellulose, hemicellulose, and lignin. It has been estimated that 20–70% of the ruminant feed is composed of the cellulose and hemicellulose [49]. The most abundant carbohydrate in plant cell wall is the cellulose which makes up to 40% of the plant cell wall. The microbial cellulolytic enzymes have the capability to digest the β-1,4 links present inside the cellulose, glucose molecules [50] (**Figure 3**).

3.4 Mechanism of action of probiotic yeast in the lower gut

The lower gut microbial population is affected by dietary supplementation of the probiotic yeast. The probiotics provide a desirable microbial balance due to shift in the balance of friendly and pathogenic microbiota. The GIT having healthy microbial populations are often related with improved host performance and its immune system. In the lower gut, the pathogenic microbial species reduces due to the production of the antimicrobial material (bacteriocin) and the attachment of the friendly microbes to the gut wall, via the competitive exclusive method. The most common modulation of the GIT microflora is provided by probiotics [51].

4. Modern methods to understand and develop fibrolytic probiotics for ruminants

Latest researches have improved our understanding related to the mode of action of probiotic yeast inside the rumen. Well-designed animal studies have verified that target-specific probiotic strains have health and production benefits in the ruminants. These studies have made the livestock industry to accept and understand the probiotic concept [52]. On the other hand, current probiotic has not been chosen for definite purposes in the animal feed. Therefore, some unique molecular methods are needed for selection and characterization of target-specific probiotic strains [53]. It has been noted that during stress conditions, some portion

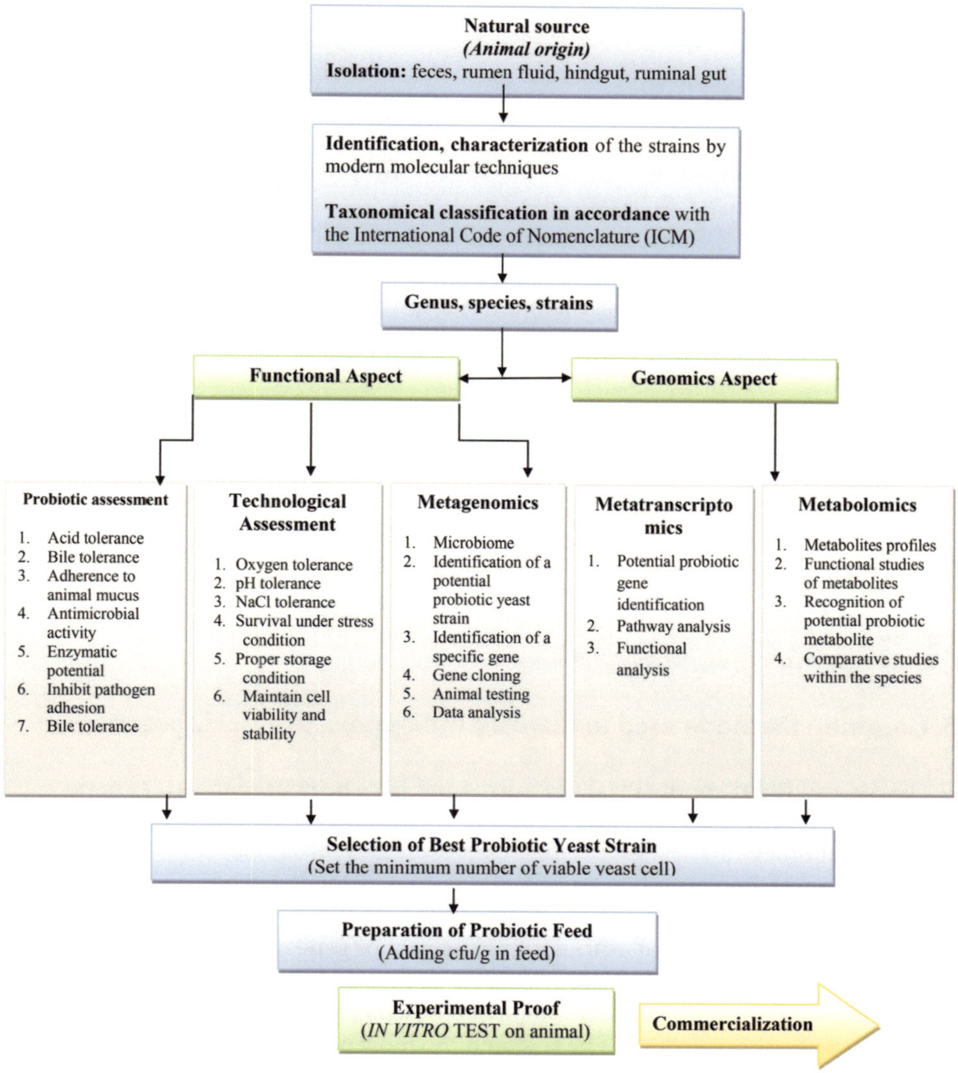

Figure 4.
Probiotic preparation: general steps for the isolation and characterization of probiotic yeast strains for local animal breed.

of the live probiotic microbial strain enters in the dormant but metabolically active state called viable but nonculturable (VBNC) state. These microbial cells have an ability to replicate when acclimated to a favorable condition inside the host [54]. Uses of molecular techniques have changed the study of the rumen ecosystem. First is the PCR which is more sensitive than growth on traditional selective media in determining small differences in population sizes in response to dietary changes or upon the inclusion of an additive to the diet and thus may identify changes or shifts within levels of the microbial population which may have been previously overlooked [55] (**Figure 4**).

In response to various feeding sources, changes within the microbial population can be studied by DNA fingerprinting (DGGE, TTGE, and TGGE). Probiotic can be classified into three different types, like mono-probiotic, poly probiotics, and combined probiotics depending on the probiotic strain function [55] (**Figure 5**).

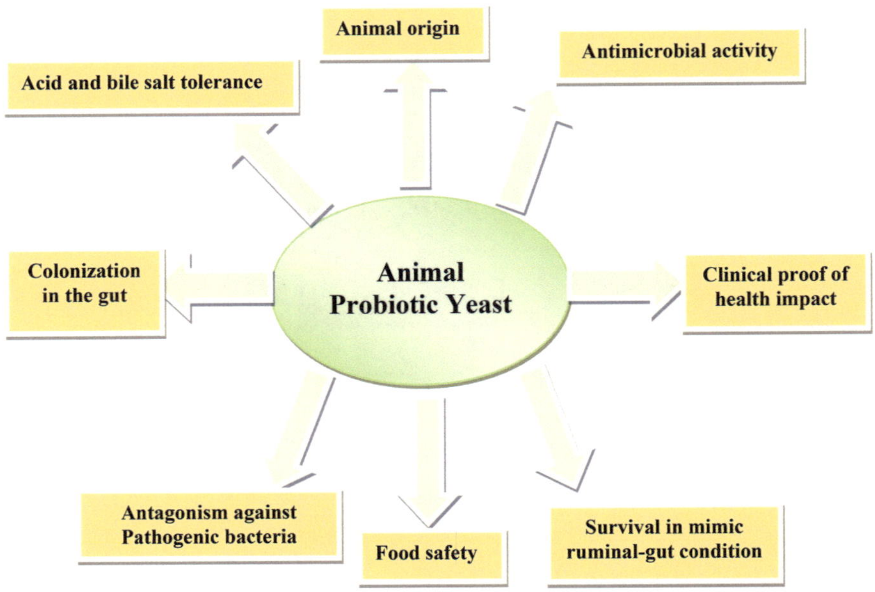

Figure 5.
Potential characteristics of typical animal probiotic yeast.

5. Common methods used to identify indigenous probiotic yeast

Yeasts and fungi are the ideal organisms and have been used in vast genetic studies and comparative genomic studies in eukaryotes because of their small and compact genomes.

We have sketched sampling approaches and finalized the protocols that will guide researchers in identifying the most ideal probiotics for animal use. Livestock is under increasing threat of antimicrobial resistance genes; therefore, continued optimization of protocols is urgently needed so that these threats can be reduced through the use of probiotics. Two sequence-based methods are commonly used for the identification of yeast. The first and the most common method used for the identification is PCR amplification of internal transcribed spacer (ITS) of nuclear ribosomal variable region that has been recognized as the universal barcode for the identification of fungi. The second and the advanced approach to identify fungal species or strains is shotgun metagenomics [56]. Microbes are very vital to life present on the earth. Their significance is increasing day by day as their beneficiary potential has been recognized in the field of health and medicine. There are two methods which have been utilized till now for the identification of the microorganisms present in microbial community.

- Culture-dependent method
- Culture-independent method

Both approaches have their own significance. Culture-based methods are considered effective for the morphological, physiological, and functional characterizations of a particular strain, while culture-independent technology is preferred to unravel the microbial diversity along with genomic and genetic identification of microbial communities. Studies have also indicated that there is a loss of 99% microbes in the laboratory-dependent culturing methods. Culturing-independent method has been recognized as an effective and efficient method to isolate the DNA of a number of microbes from an environmental sample which seems impossible using the cultural methods. The linkage of culture-dependent and culture-independent data has been recognized as a crucial step for the identification of probiotics [57]. For identification of the potential probiotic strains, researchers should use the latest molecular methods, and the probiotic strains should be deposited in some recognized microbial culture collection. Proteomics and metabolomics may also be used for choosing the best yeast species [58]. By utilizing strain's proteome and metabolome, which are argued to yield a positive influence upon ruminal fermentation, it may be possible to identify specific traits, characteristics, and secondary growth metabolites that play a potential role to enhance the growth of target-specific microorganisms inside the rumen. Even accounting for the potential bias of latest molecular methods, it is obvious that these methods are the dominant tools recently accessible for monitoring the gut for bacterial diversity of dairy animals and developing new yeast strain [59]. Extensive use of molecular methodologies may give insights into the new era where such microbial studies are no longer limited to a handful of laboratories with an abundance of funding and labor. It is noted that the specific yeast strains of known origin act more precisely and efficiently as compared to the yeast strain obtained from any unknown origin [60]. As we note all ruminates live in different parts of the world; therefore, upon the ruminal fermentation different yeast strains may exhibit markedly different effects. Therefore, we should identify new yeast strains for getting best results on the rumen fermentation. Uses of molecular techniques have changed the study of the rumen ecosystem. First is the PCR which is more sensitive than growth on traditional selective media in determining small differences in population sizes in response to dietary changes or upon the inclusion of an additive to the diet and thus may identify changes or shifts within levels of the microbial population which may have been previously overlooked. In response to various feeding sources, changes within the microbial population can be studied by DNA fingerprinting (DGGE, TTGE, and TGGE). To select best yeast strains, proteomics and metabolomics may also be used. By characterizing the proteome and metabolome of microbial isolates endowed with the ability to have a positive impact on the rumen fermentation, it may be possible to identify specific traits, characteristics, and secondary growth metabolites which play genuine role in the improvement of the growth of some important microbial species [61] (**Figure 6**).

5.1 Culture-dependent techniques

Cultural approach is the widely used method in microbiology to grow a microbe in a laboratory. Sampling is the basic and the crucial step for the identification of the indigenous probiotic yeast. The second step is isolation of the pure yeast strain under laboratory conditions which requires a series of inoculation steps of the microbes on the selective media. After purification of the yeast isolate on the OGA media, the biochemical tests are performed to identify the distinct features of the pure isolates. Morphological features of the isolate are determined by using electron microscope. The next step is the molecular identification of the yeast via 18S rRNA gene sequencing. The probiotic characterization is usually performed according to the standards defined by the WHO [62]. The best probiotic strain is retrieved among all the selected potential candidates, and in vivo experiments are performed using an animal model. After functional testing, all technological and safety measures are accessed, and the probiotic yeast strain is ready for probiotic product and packaging [63].

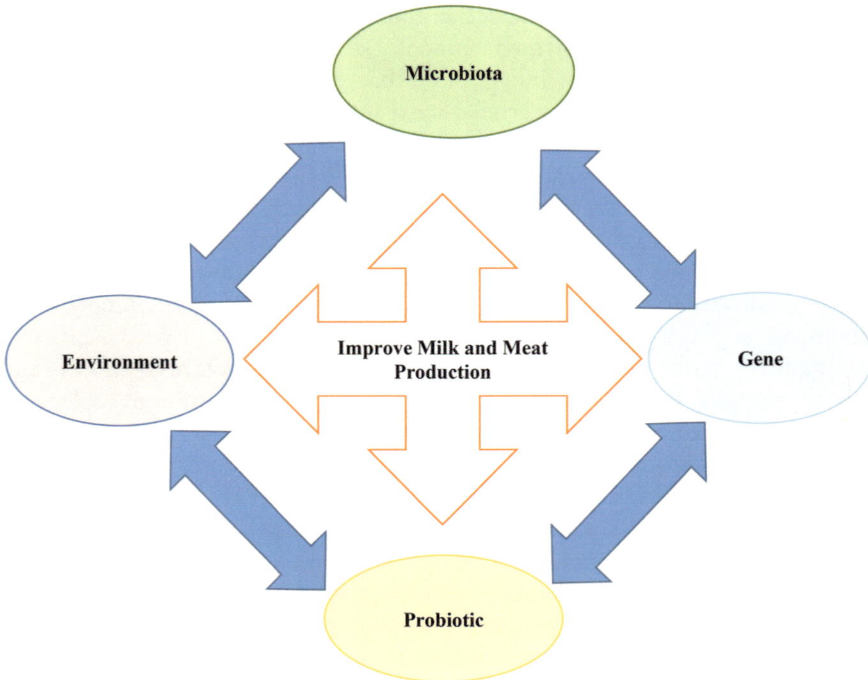

Figure 6.
Interlinked factors involved in the application of probiotic in the ruminant nutrition.

5.2 Culture-independent techniques

The use of omics approach has been emphasized to study the microbiome of microbes. To identify the potential probiotic strains among the microbial community present in any environment, it is very important to identify all the microorganisms in microbiota and determine their structural and functional differences at genomic level. Below are the currently available omics approaches for the identification, screening, and selection of probiotic strains of indigenous yeast [64] (**Figure 7**).

5.2.1 18S amplicon sequencing

Amplicon sequencing refers to the sequencing of a specific fragment of interest of a microbe using high-throughput sequencing technique. 18S amplicon sequencing is specifically used to determine the most prevalent fungal yeast species present in microbiota [65]. The methodologies used in the recent researches for the identification of bacterial probiotics can be applied in the recognition of indigenous probiotic yeast strains. The comparative and detailed analysis of 18S amplicon sequencing data can help the scientists in the isolation of potential probiotic after the identification of functional and structural characteristics of the indigenous yeast in microbiota. Further experiments and testing would be required to maximize the production and ability of probiotic yeast in the gut of an animal [66]. Furthermore, the 18S amplicon sequencing does not only help in the indigenous yeast identification, but it also reveals the diversity of microeukaryotes when 18S rRNA gene is sequenced [67].

5.2.2 Shotgun metagenomics

Shotgun metagenomics is one of the most advanced techniques of sequencing in which the entire microbiome of microbiota is sequenced. The data generated

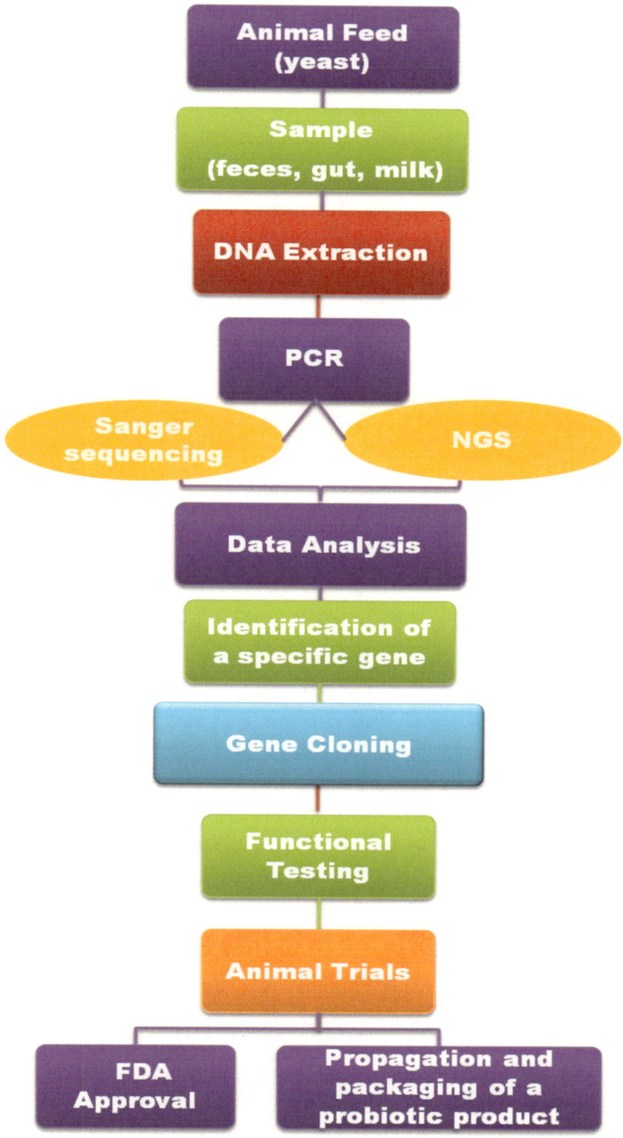

Figure 7.
Omics approaches to identify the probiotic.

using this method provides all the information about the genome of an organism [68]. Metagenomics information unravels the composition of microbial community and also indicates the genes, their functions, and associated genetic pathways. The identification of the indigenous yeast and their probiotic potential and capabilities can also be determined using the metagenomics data. Their relationship within the microbial community and their effect on the host can also be studied on the basis of the retrieved information [69].

5.2.3 Metatranscriptomics

Scientists and researchers are using metatrancriptomics to study and analyze the expression profiles of mRNA in a microbial community. The identification of genes, genetic pathways and their regulation, host-microbe interaction, and the symbiotic relation among microbes can easily be determined by using the mRNA expression data. Metatranscriptome approach can be pursued in the identification of indigenous probiotic yeast within the microbiota of an animal. For this purpose the sampling methods and molecular techniques should be improved [70].

5.2.4 Metabolomics

Metabolomics refers to the study of the metabolites or final cellular products. This is also considered one of the useful and efficient methods for the identification of probiotic potential of a microorganism within a microbiota of an animal or selected biological sample [71]. Indigenous probiotic potential of yeast can also be determined using this technique. Studies are still needed to fully understand the function of metabolites in context of probiotic potential and other inhibitory functions of metabolic compounds. As metabolites vary in structure and function, so they could be used in the comparative studies of species and populations. A number of species with high probiotic potential could be approached using metabolomics [72].

6. Challenges in preparation of suitable probiotic yeast

- Yeast probiotics not only help to improve the performance factor of cattle, but it also enhances nutrient digestibility. However, the effectiveness of yeast-supplemented products is variable. Therefore, future studies are required to estimate the potency of these diet products as supplements for finishing beef cattle, with an objective to have healthier and productive animals without negotiating their efficiency and costs.

- The animal body is a "supraorganism" and refers to the gastrointestinal tract as a virtual organ of the human body. The ongoing research is mainly on probiotics that are used chiefly for the GI tract, whereas there is an impetus need to evaluate the progress on other regions of the body as well.

- Yeast supplementation is an effective strategy; thus, it is vital to ensure the stability and viability of yeast-supplemented diet products by developing practicable and cost-effective technologies (e.g., storage, microencapsulation, etc.), which poses marketing and technological challenges for producers at industrial level. Polysaccharides, lipids, and proteins are chiefly used for encapsulation materials in food industry. However, cost-effective production remains a challenge for production of future probiotics and formulation technologies.

- Role of yeast probiotics in combating antibiotic-associated diseases has been extensively reported through control trials and ingestion of yeast probiotics (*Saccharomyces boulardii*) and has positive therapeutic effects specifically in preventing antibiotic-associated diarrhea (ADD), but validated biomarkers for numerous target diseases are probiotic or antibiotic deficient. Therefore, in the field of probiotic investigation, the defining of validated biomarkers needs to be advanced.

- There is a dire need to understand the composition and relationship of microbial community within an animal gut for improving the production of dairy products. Advances in the high-throughput technologies, computational tools, and omics approaches give insights into the molecular and genetic potential of an organism. Studies in the omics arena are still needed to fully understand the genetic mechanisms and pathway analysis.

7. Conclusions and future research

Every living organism is different in terms of their genetic makeup. The current progresses in sequencing and functional omics techniques have delivered better understandings into the precise mechanisms underlying probiotic functionality. The emerging understanding of the animal gut microbiota allowed accurate characterization of probiotic effects on the commensal microbiota of animal in vivo. Identification of genes vital to probiotic functionality is providing scientists the capacity to genetically tailor probiotics to encounter the requirements for precise applications. The livestock sector has a larger proportion of land consumption than agriculture keeping in view both grain feed intake and grazing. This trend is expected to rise, putting pressure and competencies on land resources in the agriculture sector. Moreover, there is a high demand for quality production which Cannot be attained by traditional practices for feeding ruminants. Quality cereal feed costs high and is uneconomical for large production. Consequently, this creates an imbalance in nutrition which drastically reduces dairy production. Probiotic yeast can overcome dairy production disparity. It augments nutrient uptake and increases Immunity, overall better health and production. Utilization of probiotic yeast for health and production is influenced by many different factors including probiotic strains, age, and breed of cattle. Essentially, yeast probiotics enhance assimilation by balancing the microflora of the rumen. It facilitates fiber digestion via inducing fermentation and stabilizing high pH. Facilitating an environment that flourishes rumen microbes is one factor. Other avenues need to be explored for probiotic yeast. More probiotic yeast strains are needed to be identified. For the preparation of probiotic feed, a complete nutritional profile generation is required. Furthermore, the amino acid profile of milk produced by dairy heifers fed on yeast probiotic should be analyzed.

8. Recommendations

The recommendations are outlined as follows:

- Sampling source should be indigenous for isolation of the probiotic strains.
- The identification of the probiotic strains must be based on the international validated molecular methods.
- The identified strain name should be deposited in validated microbial culture collection.
- The probiotic as well as genetic properties of the probiotic strains should be studied. Good manufacturing practices must be applied with quality assurance and shelf-life conditions established and labeling made clear to include minimum dosage and verifiable health claims.

Author details

Shakira Ghazanfar[1*], Aayesha Riaz[2], Ghulam Muhammad Ali[1], Saima Naveed[3], Irum Arif[1], Sidra Irshad[1], Naeem Riaz[1] and Khanzadi Nazneen Manzoor[1]

1 National Institute of Genomics and Advance Biotechnology (NIGAB), NARC, Islamabad, Pakistan

2 Department of Parasitology and Microbiology, Faculty of Veterinary and Animal Sciences, PMAS-Arid Agricultural University, Pakistan

3 Animal Nutrition Department, University of Veterinary and Animal Sciences Lahore, Pakistan

*Address all correspondence to: shakira_akmal@yahoo.com

References

[1] Vohra A, Syal P, Madan A. Probiotic yeasts in livestock sector. Animal Feed Science and Technology. 2016;**219**:31-47

[2] McCann JC, Elolimy AA, Loor JJ. Rumen microbiome, probiotics, and fermentation additives. Veterinary Clinics: Food Animal Practice. 2017;**33**(3):539-553

[3] Sanders ME, Huis J. Bringing a probiotic-containing functional food to the market: microbiological, product, regulatory and labeling issues. In Lactic Acid Bacteria: Genetics, Metabolism and Applications. Dordrecht: Springer; 1999. pp. 293-315

[4] Bonatsou S et al. Evaluating the probiotic potential and technological characteristics of yeasts implicated in cv. Kalamata natural black olive fermentation. International Journal of Food Microbiology. 2018;**271**:48-59

[5] Ayala D et al. Molecular detection and quantification of viable probiotic strains in animal feedstuffs using the commercial direct fed microbial *Lactobacillus* animalis NP51 as a model. Journal of Microbiological Methods. 2018;**149**:36-43

[6] Le Thi Hong Van CK, Son HPH. In vitro assessment of potential probiotic microorganisms for application in animal feeding. Journal of Science and Technology. 2016;**54**(4A):250-258

[7] Ajithakumar H et al. Effect of prilled fat and yeast supplementation on milk production, fatty acid profile and economics of feeding in murrah buffaloes (*Bubalus bubalis*). International Journal of Current Microbiology and Applied Sciences. 2017;**6**(10):1757-1767

[8] Vyas D et al. The effects of active dried and killed dried yeast on subacute ruminal acidosis, ruminal fermentation, and nutrient digestibility in beef heifers. Journal of Animal Science. 2014;**92**(2):724-732

[9] Uyeno Y, Shigemori S, Shimosato T. Effect of probiotics/prebiotics on cattle health and productivity. Microbes and Environments. 2015;**30**(2):126-132

[10] Zoumpopoulou G, Kazou M, Alexandraki V, Angelopoulou A, Papadimitriou K, Pot B, et al. Probiotics and Prebiotics: An Overview on Recent Trends. In Probiotics and Prebiotics in Animal Health and Food Safety. Cham.: Springer; 2018. pp. 1-34

[11] Markowiak P, Śliżewska K. The role of probiotics, prebiotics and synbiotics in animal nutrition. Gut Pathogens. 2018;**10**(1):21

[12] Makkar HP, McSweeney CS, editors. Methods in gut microbial ecology for ruminants. Dordrecht, Netherlands: Springer; 2005;**10**:1-4020

[13] Dowd SE et al. Evaluation of the bacterial diversity in the feces of cattle using 16S rDNA bacterial tag-encoded FLX amplicon pyrosequencing (bTEFAP). BMC Microbiology. 2008;**8**(1):125

[14] Ghazanfar S, Azim A. Metagenomics and its application in rumen ecosystem: Potential biotechnological prospects. Pakistan Journal of Nutrition. 2009;**8**(8):1309-1315

[15] Hoseinifar SH et al. The effects of oligofructose on growth performance, survival and autochthonous intestinal microbiota of beluga (*Huso huso*) juveniles. Aquaculture Nutrition. 2011;**17**(5):498-504

[16] Reti KL et al. Effect of antimicrobial growth promoter administration on the intestinal microbiota of beef cattle. Gut Pathogens. 2013;**5**(1):8

[17] Gaggìa F, Mattarelli P, Biavati B. Probiotics and prebiotics in animal feeding for safe food production. International Journal of Food Microbiology. 2010;**141**: S15-S28

[18] Tellez G et al. Probiotics/direct fed microbials for Salmonella control in poultry. Food Research International. 2012;**45**(2):628-633

[19] Simon O, Jadamus A, Vahjen W. Probiotic feed additives-effectiveness and expected modes of action. Journal of Animal and Feed Sciences. 2001;**10**:51-68

[20] Zimmermann B, Bauer E, Mosenthin R. Pro-and prebiotics in pig nutrition-potential modulators of gut health? Journal of Animal and Feed Sciences. 2001;**10**(1):47-56

[21] Hajela N et al. Gut microbiome, gut function, and probiotics: Implications for health. Indian Journal of Gastroenterology. 2015;**34**(2): 93-107

[22] Bitencourt LL et al. Diet digestibility and performance of dairy cows supplemented with live yeast. Scientia Agricola. 2011;**68**(3):301-307

[23] Beev G, Todorova P, Tchobanova S. Yeast cultures in ruminant nutrition. Bulgarian Journal of Agricultural Science. 2007;**13**:357-374

[24] Baiomy A. Influence of live yeast culture on milk production, composition and some blood metabolites of ossimi ewes during the milking period. American Journal of Biochemistry and Molecular Biology. 2011;**1**(2):158-167

[25] Chaucheyras-Durand F, Chevaux E, Martin C, Forano E. Use of yeast probiotics in ruminants: Effects and mechanisms of action on rumen pH, fibre degradation, and microbiota according to the diet. In Probiotic in animals. Intech. 2012

[26] Campanile G et al. Effects of *Saccharomyces cerevisiae* on in vivo organic matter digestibility and milk yield in buffalo cows. Livestock Science. 2008;**114**(2-3):358-361

[27] Newbold CJ, Wallace R, McIntosh F. Mode of action of the yeast *Saccharomyces cerevisiae* as a feed additive for ruminants. British Journal of Nutrition. 1996;**76**(2): 249-261

[28] Hansen HH, El-Bordeny NE, Ebeid HM. Response of primiparous and multiparous buffaloes to yeast culture supplementation during early and mid-lactation. Animal Nutrition. 2017;**3**(4):411-418

[29] Ogbuewu I et al. Yeast (*Saccharomyces cerevisiae*) and its effect on production indices of livestock and poultry—A review. Comparative Clinical Pathology. 2018:1-9

[30] Clauss M, Hofmann RR. The digestive system of ruminants, and peculiarities of (wild) cattle. Ecology, evolution and behaviour of wild cattle: Implications for conservation. 2014:57-62.a

[31] Burns J. ASAS centennial paper: Utilization of pasture and forages by ruminants: A historical perspective. Journal of Animal Science. 2008;**86**(12):3647-3663

[32] Wahrmund J et al. Ruminal acidosis challenge impact on ruminal temperature in feedlot cattle. Journal of Animal Science. 2012;**90**(8): 2794-2801

[33] Brod D, Bolsen K, Brent B. Effect of water temperature in rumen temperature, digestion and rumen fermentation in sheep. Journal of Animal Science. 1982;**54**(1):179-182

[34] Penner G et al. Ruminant nutrition symposium: Molecular adaptation of ruminal epithelia to highly fermentable diets. Journal of Animal Science. 2011;**89**(4):1108-1119

[35] Stefańska B et al. Prevalence and consequence of subacute ruminal acidosis in Polish dairy herds. Journal of Animal Physiology and Animal Nutrition. 2017;**101**(4):694-702

[36] Russell JB, Wilson DB. Why are ruminal cellulolytic bacteria unable to digest cellulose at low pH? Journal of Dairy Science. 1996;**79**(8):1503-1509

[37] Lodemann U, Martens H. Effects of diet and osmotic pressure on Na+ transport and tissue conductance of sheep isolated rumen epithelium. Experimental Physiology. 2006;**91**(3):539-550

[38] Henderson G et al. Rumen microbial community composition varies with diet and host, but a core microbiome is found across a wide geographical range. Scientific Reports. 2015;**5**:14567

[39] Fouts DE et al. Next generation sequencing to define prokaryotic and fungal diversity in the bovine rumen. PLoS One. 2012;**7**(11):e48289

[40] Liggenstoffer AS et al. Phylogenetic diversity and community structure of anaerobic gut fungi (*Phylum neocallimastigomycota*) in ruminant and non-ruminant herbivores. The ISME Journal. 2010;**4**(10):1225

[41] Gruninger RJ et al. Anaerobic fungi (*Phylum neocallimastigomycota*): Advances in understanding their taxonomy, life cycle, ecology, role and biotechnological potential. FEMS Microbiology Ecology. 2014;**90**(1):1-17

[42] Khan RU et al. Direct-fed microbial: Beneficial applications, modes of action and prospects as a safe tool for enhancing ruminant production and safeguarding health. International Journal of Pharmacology. 2016;**12**(3):220-231

[43] Lin B et al. Characterization of the rumen microbial community composition of buffalo breeds consuming diets typical of dairy production systems in Southern China. Animal Feed Science and Technology. 2015;**207**:75-84

[44] Rima H, Steve L, Ismail F. Antimicrobial and probiotic properties of yeasts: From fundamental to novel applications. Frontiers in Microbiology. 2012;**3**:421

[45] Galvão KN et al. Effect of feeding live yeast products to calves with failure of passive transfer on performance and patterns of antibiotic resistance in fecal *Escherichia coli*. Reproduction Nutrition Development. 2005;**45**(4):427-440

[46] Pinloche E et al. The effects of a probiotic yeast on the bacterial diversity and population structure in the rumen of cattle. PLoS One. 2013;**8**(7):e67824

[47] Cebra JJ. Influences of microbiota on intestinal immune system development. The American Journal of Clinical Nutrition. 1999;**69**(5):1046s-1051s

[48] Kumar S et al. Associative patterns among anaerobic fungi, methanogenic archaea, and bacterial communities in response to changes in diet and age in the rumen of dairy cows. Frontiers in Microbiology. 2015;**6**:781

[49] Hungate R. The rumen microbial ecosystem. Annual Review of Ecology and Systematics. 1975;**6**(1):39-66

[50] Flint HJ et al. Polysaccharide utilization by gut bacteria: Potential for new insights from genomic analysis. Nature Reviews Microbiology. 2008;**6**(2):121

[51] Oelschlaeger TA. Mechanisms of probiotic actions–A review. International Journal of Medical Microbiology. 2010;**300**(1):57-62

[52] AlZahal O et al. Factors influencing ruminal bacterial community diversity and composition and microbial fibrolytic enzyme abundance in lactating dairy cows with a focus on the role of active dry yeast. Journal of Dairy Science. 2017;**100**(6):4377-4393

[53] Gueimonde M, Salminen S. New methods for selecting and evaluating probiotics. Digestive and Liver Disease. 2006;**38**:S242-S247

[54] Davis C. Enumeration of probiotic strains: Review of culture-dependent and alternative techniques to quantify viable bacteria. Journal of Microbiological Methods. 2014;**103**:9-17

[55] Maldonado N et al. Effect of milk fermented with lactic acid bacteria on diarrheal incidence, growth performance and microbiological and blood profiles of newborn dairy calves. Probiotics and Antimicrobial Proteins. 2018;**10**(4):668-676

[56] Donovan PD et al. Identification of fungi in shotgun metagenomics datasets. PLoS One. 2018;**13**(2):e0192898

[57] Akinbowale OL, Peng H, Barton MD. Antimicrobial resistance in bacteria isolated from aquaculture sources in Australia. Journal of Applied Microbiology. 2006;**100**(5):1103-1113

[58] de Melo Pereira GV et al. How to select a probiotic? A review and update of methods and criteria. Biotechnology Advances. 2018;**36**(8):2060-2076

[59] Islam M, Lee S-S. Recent application technologies of rumen microbiome is the key to enhance feed fermentation. Journal of Life Science. 2018;**28**(10):1244-1253

[60] Bagheripoor-Fallah N et al. Comparison of molecular techniques with other methods for identification and enumeration of probiotics in fermented milk products. Critical Reviews in Food Science and Nutrition. 2015;**55**(3):396-413

[61] Yadav R, Shukla P. An overview of advanced technologies for selection of probiotics and their expediency: A review. Critical Reviews in Food Science and Nutrition. 2017;**57**(15):3233-3242

[62] Panda SH, Goli JK, Das S. Production, optimization and probiotic characterization of potential lactic acid bacteria producing siderophores. AIMS Microbiology. 2017;**3**(1):88-107

[63] Silvestri G et al. Investigation of the microbial ecology of Ciauscolo, a traditional Italian salami, by culture-dependent techniques and PCR-DGGE. Meat Science. 2007;**77**(3):413-423

[64] Greppi A et al. Determination of yeast diversity in ogi, mawè, gowé and tchoukoutou by using culture-dependent and-independent methods. International Journal of Food Microbiology. 2013;**165**(2):84-88

[65] He J-Z et al. Microbial composition and diversity of an upland red soil under long-term fertilization treatments as revealed by culture-dependent and culture-independent approaches. Journal of Soils and Sediments. 2008;**8**(5):349-358

[66] Rebollar EA et al. Using "omics" and integrated multi-omics approaches to guide probiotic selection to mitigate chytridiomycosis and other emerging

infectious diseases. Frontiers in Microbiology. 2016;**7**:68

[67] Findley K et al. Topographic diversity of fungal and bacterial communities in human skin. Nature. 2013;**498**(7454):367

[68] Ghazanfar S et al. Metagenomics and its application in soil microbial community studies: Biotechnological prospects. Journal of Animal & Plant Sciences. 2010;**6**(2):611-622

[69] Lindahl BD et al. Fungal community analysis by high-throughput sequencing of amplified markers–A user's guide. New Phytologist. 2013;**199**(1):288-299

[70] Qin J et al. A human gut microbial gene catalogue established by metagenomic sequencing. Nature. 2010;**464**(7285):59

[71] Jung JY et al. Metatranscriptomic analysis of lactic acid bacterial gene expression during kimchi fermentation. International Journal of Food Microbiology. 2013;**163**(2-3):171-179

[72] Gosalbes MJ et al. Metatranscriptomic approach to analyze the functional human gut microbiota. PLoS One. 2011;**6**(3):e17447

Chapter 3

Yeasts as Dietary Additives to Manipulate Ruminal Fermentation: Effect on Nutrient Utilization and Productive Performance of Ruminants

Oscar Ruiz Barrera, Jaime Salinas-Chavira and Yamicela Castillo Castillo

Abstract

There is considerable interest in the use of microbial additives such as yeasts in the nutrition of ruminants. The prohibition of the antibiotics as growth promoters in animal feeds increased the interest to investigate the effects of yeasts as natural additives on the gastrointestinal ecosystem and animal productive behavior. The effect of yeast-based preparations on the rumen environment and on the growth performance of ruminants has been well documented and has generated considerable scientific attention in the last two decades. However, the precise action modes by which the yeast cultures improve nutrient utilization and livestock production are still under study. Therefore, the objective of this chapter is to deepen into the action mechanisms of the yeasts at the ruminal level and at the productive level for their use as additives in animal feeding.

Keywords: ruminants, probiotics, natural additives, feeding, growth

1. Introduction

The yeasts are not part of the ruminal ecosystem, and their presence is mainly due to the ingestion in feeds and water. Marrero [1] and Castillo-Castillo et al. [2] showed that supplementing ruminant feeds rich in yeasts, they survived for longer time in the rumen and improved the conditions that favored the dry matter (DM) use by microorganisms that inhabit in it. These results corroborate the approach made by Galves [3] that when certain allochthonous microorganisms are deposited in a new habitat with nutrients, they survive and are able to use part of the resources of the environment in which they were deposited; in this case, the yeasts use the little oxygen existing in rumen and favor the conditions of anaerobiosis [4] that facilitate or potentiate the growth of other anaerobic microorganisms as the cellulolytic bacteria.

Research reports where yeasts are a natural alternative to manipulate ruminal microbial fermentation and animal productivity are shown below. Yeasts have shown to improve the digestibility of DM and neutral detergent fiber (NDF) [5], feed consumption [6], milk production [7], and live weight gain [8]. However, not all yeast cultures have been shown to modify ruminal metabolism or improve animal productivity [9, 10]. These inconsistencies could be related to the type of yeast strain used [11], the specificity of the different commercial additives [12], or to the diet composition [13]. The objective of this review was to deepen into the mechanisms of action of the yeasts as well as their effects at the ruminal level and at a productive level for their use as animal feed additives.

2. Yeasts

Yeasts are unicellular microorganisms that ferment carbohydrates, and they are reproduced by budding. Most commercial yeast-based products contain a mixture of varying proportions of living cells of *Saccharomyces cerevisiae* and dead cells. Products with a predominance of living cells are sold as live yeasts, while those containing more dead cells with the growth medium are sold as yeast cultures [14]. Examples include Yea-SACC (Alltech Inc.), Levucell SC-20 (Lallemand Animal Nutrition), and Yeast Cultivation Diamond V (Diamond V, Mills Inc.). Yeast cultures are foods generally considered as safe (GRAS) denomination given by the Food and Drug Administration (FDA) (USA).

3. Mechanisms of action of yeasts in the rumen

One of the proposed action modes is that living yeasts through their aerobic respiration allow the elimination of the small percentage of oxygen (1%) that enters to the rumen when the animal ingests their feeds, thus facilitating the growth of the most anaerobic microorganisms as cellulolytic bacteria and fungi [4, 15].

Another proposed mechanism of action is that yeast cultures provide vitamins (specifically thiamin), glucans, mannano-proteins, and organic acids, which stimulate the growth of microorganisms that digest fiber and use lactic acid [16–18].

An additional effect is that yeast cultures are rich in organic acids (mainly malic acid) that stimulate the growth of *Selenomonas ruminantium*. This ruminal bacterium consumes the lactic acid produced in the rumen and therefore contributes to the stabilization of the pH in rumen, which favors the growth of cellulolytic microorganisms [17].

Yeasts also produce changes in the bacterial flora by competition and growth stimulation, increasing the growth, and activity of the acetogenic populations that compete with the methanogenic ones by the use of the metabolic hydrogen [16]. This decrease the energy losses in the animal caused the methane formed in rumen, which decreases the negative effect of this greenhouse gas on the environment [19].

4. Effect of the addition of yeasts in the ruminal fermentation

Yeast cultures based on *Saccharomyces cerevisiae* have been widely used in the diet of ruminants to improve digestibility and DM utilization [14].

The yeast products available in the market vary widely depending on the strain of *S. cerevisiae* used and the number and viability of the cells. Some products guarantee a high number of live yeast cells, while other products are sold as yeast cultures, which contain living cells and the medium where they grew [14].

Interestingly, it has been observed that not all strains of *S. cerevisiae* are capable to stimulate digestion in the rumen [11, 12]. For example, yeast culture "Diamond-VXP" and "A-Max Concentrate" generated different values of ruminal pH and molar concentration of total and individual VFA [12]. These differences were not related to the number of viable cells in the preparation or to the differences in metabolic activity [11].

In vitro and in vivo studies found no effect of yeasts on ruminal pH [4, 20–24]. However, results where pH decreased were reported by Williams [6] when they supplemented *S. cerevisiae* (10 g/d) in steers consuming barley hay. Lynch and Martin [25] also found a decrease in pH at adequate values for ruminal cellulolysis when they studied the in vitro effect of a *S. cerevisiae* culture on the fermentation of Bermuda hay and alfalfa hay.

On the other hand, regarding to the concentration of ammonia-nitrogen ($N\text{-}NH_3$), Lila et al. [22] and Erasmus et al. [20] showed that the inclusion of yeast does not affect the levels of this compound. Contrary to the above, Lattimer et al. [21] reported a decrease in the $N\text{-}NH_3$ concentration when they evaluated the effect of a yeast culture on the in vitro fermentation of a high fiber diet. Also, Moallem et al. [26] reported a decrease in ruminal $N\text{-}NH_3$ from dairy cows supplemented with yeast.

Other effects of yeasts include increase in metabolites as VFA [12, 18], decrease in lactic acid concentration [22], reduction of methane production [22, 25], increase in growth of cellulolytic bacteria and fungi [4, 16, 22] as well as acetogenic bacteria [16], and increase in fiber degradability [12, 22].

5. Use of yeasts in animal feeding

The use of feed additives is important in the feeding of ruminants. Yeast proteins have a high nutritional value, characterized by a balanced amino acid profile with a high content of lysine and threonine, which gives it an extraordinary potential for use as a supplement to animal diets, since these could be deficient in these amino acids [27].

The yeast of *Saccharomyces cerevisiae* as an additive in animal nutrition has been extensively investigated; however, the results obtained are variable and not very repeatable, possibly due to the great diversity of diets offered to the animals in study, the different strains of yeasts, and the different doses supplied to the animals. It is pointed out that *S. cerevisiae* increases feed consumption, milk production, feed conversion, and daily gain of weight, in response to increases in the amount and activity of the total anaerobic and cellulolytic bacteria that modify the concentration of volatile fatty acids, ruminal pH, and ammonia-nitrogen; however, the results are not consistent, so it is recommended to differentiate *S. cerevisiae* yeast strains that promote the use of the neutral detergent fiber of the ration [28].

Baiomy [29], in a study carried out with lactating sheep, mentioned that supplementation with live yeasts of *S. cerevisiae* has a significant effect on the development and metabolism of animals during the lactation period. In view of the above, it is recommended to include live yeast (Yea Sacc1026) in the animal diet in an amount of 6 g $animal^{-1}$ day^{-1}. On the other hand, Sotillo et al. [30] in dairy goats found that the addition to the diet of 0.08 g kg^{-1} of dry matter of the additive Yea-Sacc® TS (*S. cerevisiae*) causes a 7% increase in milk production and an increase in the percentage of fat in it. In turn, there is an increase in the level of urea in milk and an improvement in body condition. There was also a decrease in somatic cell count values, indicative of a better health status of the animals. It is necessary to consider that the effects of the yeasts can be variable, depending on several factors related to the animal (species, physiological stage, consumption, etc.) and/or diet (composition of the diet, mode of distribution, etc.) [31, 32]. However, the concentration of viable cells, the type of yeast, and the used dose are also of great importance in this variability [33]. In this regard, little research has been conducted to determine the effects of different doses of the microbial additive, and the doses used differ only in a narrow range, from 2 to 5 times [33, 34].

6. Other non-*Saccharomyces* strains of yeasts with potential commercial use as probiotics

A joint project carried out by Cuban and Mexican researchers has developed additives based on native yeasts adapted to their local conditions, showing a good potential to be utilized as growth enhancers in ruminants and could be economically competitive in the international market. Several studies have been conducted to examine the potential use of these non-saccharomyces yeasts on animal nutrition [35, 36]. Additionally, Marrero et al. [37] studied the effects of the addition of two strains, Levazoot 15 (*Candida norvegensis*) and Levica 25 (*Candida tropicalis*), and found that both yeasts stimulated ruminal fermentation of oat straw and alfalfa, although it was better when the Levazoot 15 was inoculated. In recent study, Castillo-Castillo et al. [2] demonstrated the fermentative capacity of Levazoot 15, which showed greatest gas production than the yeast-free control and positively affected the in vitro ruminal fermentation parameters of alfalfa and oat straw. Based on these results, the Levazoot 15 yeast strain could be potentially used as an additive for ruminants consuming high-fiber diets. In another study, Ruiz et al. [38] showed that the same strain of yeast did not affect the ruminal cellulolytic bacterial counts. However, the treatment with yeast cultures positively influenced the cellulolytic fungal populations in rumen after 4 h of incubation. Methane production did not exhibit any trends across the fermentation times. A significant reduction in methane production was only observed at 8 h by the yeast treatment; at other time points, there were noticeable numerical decreases, although not statistically significance. In addition, Levazoot 15 strain also increased volatile fatty acid (VFA) concentration such as acetic, propionic, butyric, valeric, and isovaleric acids and enhanced the in vitro dry matter digestibility (IVDMD). In accordance, Ando et al. [39] with different strains of *Candida utilis* studied the in vitro degradation of grain and forage; the results showed that the microorganisms not only increased fibers degradability but also improved the utilization of the lipids. Finally, in a related study reported by Angulo-Montoya et al. [40], *C. norvegensis* Levazoot 15 strain preferred glucose as an energy source than other carbohydrates such as sucrose and lactose for its growth. In this study, only manganese was used as trace element, and the addition of vitamins in the culture medium was not required. This yeast used tryptone as a nitrogen source and did not denote sodium requirements.

7. Conclusions

The results in the use of yeast as feed additives are not conclusive; however, in rumen, they stimulate the growth and activity of total and cellulolytic bacteria, improving fiber digestion, synthesis of microbial protein, enhances feed intake and growth performance of ruminants. Yeasts also use ruminal oxygen, facilitating the growth of obligate anaerobes. In addition, yeasts may stimulate the bacteria that consume the lactic acid produced in rumen and may contribute to modulate the pH in rumen, reducing the risks of acidosis, and it can contribute significantly to the reduction of production of methane in the rumen.

Author details

Oscar Ruiz Barrera[1], Jaime Salinas-Chavira[2] and Yamicela Castillo Castillo[1*]

1 Facultad de Zootecnia de la Universidad Autónoma de Chihuahua, Mexico

2 Facultad de Medicina Veterinaria y Zootecnia de la Universidad Autónoma de Tamaulipas, Mexico

*Address all correspondence to: ycastillo75@yahoo.com

References

[1] Marrero Y. Las levaduras como mejoradoras de la fermentación ruminal de dietas con alto contenido de fibra [tesis doctoral]. La Habana, Cuba: Instituto de Ciencia Animal; 2005

[2] Castillo-Castillo Y, Ruiz-Barrera O, Burrola-Barraza ME, Marrero-Rodriguez Y, Salinas-Chavira J, Angulo-Montoya C, et al. Isolation and characterization of yeasts from fermented apple bagasse as additives for ruminant feeding. Brazilian Journal of Microbiology. 2016;**47**:889-895

[3] Galves G. Características generales de las principales familias de microorganismos. 2005. Available from: http://www.cellsalive.com

[4] Newbold CJ, Wallace RJ, Mc Intosh FM. Mode of action of the yeast *Saccharomyces cerevisiae* as a feed additive for ruminants. British Journal of Nutrition. 1996;**96**:249-261

[5] Plata PF, Mendoza MGD, Barcena-Gama JR, Gonzalez MS. Effect of a yeast culture (*Saccharomyces cerevisiae*) on neutral detergent fiber digestion in steers fed oat straw based diets. Animal Feed Science and Technology. 1994;**49**:203-210

[6] Williams AG. The biochemical activities and importance of the ciliated protozoa in the rumen ecosystem. In: Coombs GH, North MJ, editors. Biochemical Protozoology. London. Washington: Taylor & Francis Group; 1991. pp. 61-79

[7] Dann HM, Prockley JR, McCoy GC, Hutjens MF, Garrett JE. Effects of yeast cultures (*Saccharomyces cerevisiae*) on prepartum intake and postpartum intake and milk production of Jersey cows. Journal of Dairy Science. 2000;**83**:123-127

[8] Drennan M. Effect of Yea Sacc 1026 on feed intake and performance of finishing bulls. In: Supplement to the Proceedings of Alltech's 6th Annual Symposium. Nicholasville, KY: Alltech Technical Publications; 1990. p. 495

[9] Cabrera EJI, Mendoza MGD, Aranda IE, Garcia- Bojalil C, Barcena GR, Ramos JJ. *Saccharomyces cerevisiae* and nitrogenous supplementation in growing steers grazing tropical pastures. Animal Feed Science and Technology. 2000;**83**:49-55

[10] García CCG, Mendoza MGD, Gonzalez MS, Cobos PM, Ortega ME, Ramirez LR. Effect of a yeast cultura (*Saccharomyces cerevisiae*) and monensin on ruminal fermentation and digestión in sheep. Animal Feed Science and Technology. 2000;**83**:165-170

[11] Newbold CJ, Wallace RJ, Chen XB, McIntosh FM. Different strains of *Saccharomyces cerevisiae* differ in their effects on ruminal bacterial nummers in vitro and in sheep. Journal of Animal Science. 1995;**73**:1811-1818

[12] Miller-Webster T, Hoover WH, Holt M. Influence of yeast culture on ruminal microbial metabolism in continuous culture. Journal of Dairy Science. 2002;**85**:2009-2014

[13] Adams AL, Harris B, Van Horn HH, Wilcox CJ. Effects of varing forage types on milk production responses to whole cottonseed, tallow, and yeast. Journal of Dairy Science. 1995;**78**:573-581

[14] Newbold CJ, Rode LM. Dietary additives to control methanogenesis in the rumen. International Congress Series. 2006;**1293**:138-147

[15] Rose AH. Yeast culture a microoganism for all species: A theoretical look at its mode of action. In: Proceedings Alltechs Third Annual Symposium; Biotechnology in the Feed

Industry; Nicholasville, Kentuki, USA; 1987

[16] Chaucheyras F, Fonty G, Bertin G, Gouet P. Effects of live *Saccharomyce cerevisiae* cells on zoospore germination, growth, and cellulolytic activity of the rumen anaerobic fungus, *Neocallimastix frontalis* MCH 3. Current Microbiology. 1995;**31**:201

[17] Nisbet DJ, Martin SA. The effect of *Saccharomyce cerevisiae* culture on lactate utilization by the ruminal bacterium *Selenomonas ruminantium*. Journal of Animal Science. 1991;**69**:4628

[18] Oeztuerk H, Schroeder B, Beyerbach M, Breves G. Influence of living and autoclaved yeasts of *Saccharomyces boulardii* on in vitro ruminal microbial metabolism. Journal of Dairy Science. 2005;**88**:25-2600

[19] Gamo Y, Koyama A, Zhou X, Chetra S, Santoso B, Kobayashi T, et al. Effects of monensin, nisin, probiotics and/o beta 1-4 galacto-oligosaccharide on in vitro rumen methane production. In: Global Perspective in Livestock Waste Management Proceedings of the Fourth International Livestock-Waste Management Symposium and Technology Expo; Penang, Malaysia; 19-23 May; 2002. pp. 161-163

[20] Erasmus LJ, Robinson PH, Ahmadi A, Hinders R, Garrett JE. Influence of prepartum and postpartum supplementation of a yeast culture and monensin, or both, on ruminal fermentation and performance of multiparous dairy cows. Animal Feed Science and Technology. 2005;**122**:219-239

[21] Lattimer JM, Cooper SR, Freeman DW, Lalman DL. Effect of yeast culture on in vitro fermentation of a high-concentrate or high-fiber diet using equine fecal inoculums in a daisy II incubator. Journal of Animal Science. 2007;**85**:2484-2491

[22] Lila ZA, Mohammed N, Yasui T, Kurokawa Y, Kanda S, Itabashi H. Effects of a twin strain of *Saccharomyces cerevisiae* live cells on mixed ruminal microorganism fermentation in *vitro*. Journal of Animal Science. 2004;**82**:1847-1854

[23] Longuski RA, Ying Y, Allen MS. Yeast culture supplementation prevented milk fat depression by a short-term dietary challenge with fermentable starch. Journal of Dairy Science. 2009;**92**:160-167

[24] Olson KC, Caton JS, Kirby DR, Norton PL. Influence of yeast culture supplementation and advancing season on steers grazing mixed-grass prairie in the northern great plains: II. Ruminal fermentation, site of digestion, and microbial efficiency. Journal of Animal Science. 1994;**72**:2158-2170

[25] Lynch HA, Martin SA. Effects of *Saccharomyces cerevisiae* culture and *Saccharomyces cerevisiae* live cells on *in vitro* mixed ruminal microorganism fermentation. Journal of Dairy Science. 2002;**85**:2603-2608

[26] Moallem U, Lehrer H, Livshitz L, Zachut M, Yakoby S. The effects of live yeast supplementation to dairy cows during the hot season on production feed efficiency, and digestibility. Journal of Dairy Science. 2009;**92**:343-351

[27] Gutiérrez RL, Gómez AJ. Determinación de proteína total de *Candida utilis* y *Sacharomyces cerevisiae* en bagazo de caña. Revista Lasallista de Investigación. 2008;**5**:61-64

[28] Arcos GJ, López R, Bernabé A, Hoffman J. La actividad microbiana en la fermentación ruminal y el efecto de la adición de *Saccharomyces cerevisiae*. Temas de Ciencia y tecnología. 2007;**11**:51-62

[29] Baiomy AA. Influence of yeast culture on milk production,

composition and some blood metabolites of ossimi ewes during the milking period. American Journal of Biochemistry and Molecular Biology. 2011;**1**:158-167

[30] Sotillo MJ, Gutiérrez PC, Carrizosa DJA. Ensayos para la investigación: Importancia del control lechero caprino. Revista electrónica de Veterinaria. 2009;**10**:1-9

[31] Erasmus LJ, Botha PM, Kistner A. Effect of yeast culture supplement on production, rumen fermentation, and duodenal nitrogen flow in dairy cows. Journal of Dairy Science. 1992;**75**:3056-3065

[32] Yoon IK, Stern MD. Influence of various levels of *Lactobacillus acidophilus* supplementation of fermentation by rumen microorganisms in continuous culture. In: Proceeding of 21st Biennial Conference on Rumen Function; Chicago, IL; 1991. pp. 35

[33] Fallon RJ, Earley B. Effects of Yea-Sacc®1026 inclusion on the performance of finishing bulls offered an all concentrate diet. In: Proceedings of the 20th Annual Symposium, Nutritional Biotechnology in the Feed and Food Industries (Suppl. 1); Lexington, KY, USA; May 24-26; 2004. pp. 75

[34] Wohlt JE, Finkelstein AD, Chung CH. Yeast culture to improve intake, nutrient digestibility, and performance by dairy cattle during early lactation. Journal of Dairy Science. 1991;**74**:1395-1400

[35] Marrero Y, CastilloY BE, Lovaina T, Rosa CA, Ruiz O, González E, et al. Morphological, biochemical, and molecular identification of the yeast Levica 25: A potential ruminal microbial additive. Global Veterinaria. 2011;**7**:60-65

[36] Marrero Y, Castillo Y, Burrola E, Lobaina T, Rosa CA, Ruiz O, et al. Identification of Levica yeast: As potencial ruminal microbial additive. Czech Journal of Animal Science. 2013;**58**:460-469

[37] Marrero Y, Castillo Y, Ruiz-Barrera O, Burrola E, Angulo C. Feeding of yeast (Candida spp.) improves in vitro ruminal fermentation of fibrous substrates. Journal of Integrative Agriculture. 2015;**14**:514-519

[38] Ruiz O, Castillo Y, Arzola C, Burrola E, Salinas J, Corral A, et al. Effects of *Candida norvegensis* live cells on *in vitro* oat straw rumen fermentation. Asian-Australasian Journal of Animal Sciences. 2016;**29**:211-218

[39] Ando S, Nishiguchi Y, Hayasaka K, Iefuji H, Takahashi J. Effects of *Candida utilis* treatment on the nutrient value of rice bran and the effect of *Candida utilis* on the degradation of forages *In vitro*. Asian-Australasian Journal of Animal Sciences. 2006;**19**:806

[40] Angulo-Montoya C, Ruiz-Barrera O, Castillo-Castillo Y, Marrero-Rodriguez Y, Elias-Iglesias A, Estrada-Angulo A, et al. Growth of *Candida norvegensis* with different energy, nitrogen, vitamin, and micromineral sources. Brazilian Journal of Microbiology. 2018. Published online (in press)

Section 3

Food Industry

Chapter 4

Wild Yeast and Lactic Acid Bacteria of Wine

Imma Andorrà, Gemma Miró, Noelia Espligares, Ana Maria Mislata, Miquel Puxeu and Raúl Ferrer-Gallego

Abstract

Wine is an ancient and popular alcoholic beverage made from fermented grapes. Different yeasts and bacteria strains produce different styles of wines. Over time, the inoculation of *Saccharomyces cerevisiae* strains to produce wine has been the common practice in the wine industry, and the other species of yeasts have been considered undesirable for the alcoholic fermentation. However, in the last decades, the use of wild or indigenous yeasts and lactic acid bacteria strains has significantly increased. Wild yeasts and lactic acid bacteria are interesting microorganisms that contribute to differentiate the wine character of a region. The production of wines by spontaneous or inoculated fermentations by selected wild microorganisms may be an interesting tool to improve the quality of wines. This chapter summarizes relevant aspects of these microorganisms related to this scientific field.

Keywords: biotechnology, fermentation, flavor, microbiota, *Saccharomyces*

1. Introduction

Wine is an ancient and popular alcoholic beverage made from fermented grapes. The wine quality is determined by many factors, including the climate, the soil characteristics, the grape variety and the production processes, such as the viticultural practices, the winemaking techniques and the aging period. Among these factors, the fermentations carried out during winemaking, mainly alcoholic and malolactic fermentation, strongly influence on the wine composition. Different yeasts and bacteria strains produce different styles of wines derived from the biotransformation involved in both fermentations. Generally, the alcoholic fermentation (AF) is conducted by yeasts which convert sugars into ethanol, carbon dioxide and other minor metabolites. On the other hand, the malolactic fermentation (MLF) is conducted by lactic acid bacteria (LAB), which mainly convert malic acid into lactic acid and carbon dioxide. These metabolic processes are complex and sophisticated and sometimes may induce undesirable metabolite production pathways. Accordingly, an adequate selection of the yeast and bacteria strains is an important task for winemakers.

Over time, the inoculation of *Saccharomyces cerevisiae* strains to produce wine has been the common practice in the wine industry, and the other species of yeasts have been considered undesirable for the AF. However, in the last decades, the use and the inoculation of wild, native, autochthonous or indigenous yeasts and LAB strains to conduct the AF and the MLF have been significantly increased.

The isolation, selection and inoculation of the indigenous strains are useful tools to avoid sluggish and stuck fermentations and to increase the microbial diversity, enhancing the wine character [1]. In this way, this chapter pretends to summarize the most relevant aspects of these microorganisms and showing results derived from the studies related to the wild yeast and LAB strains on the wine properties.

2. Wild microorganisms associated to wine fermentations

The biotransformation of grape juice into wine is a complex ecological and biochemical process involving the sequential development of several microbial species such as yeasts, bacteria and fungi. Yeasts are the most important micro-organisms involved in this process, being *S. cerevisiae* the main responsible of the AF. Although there are other genera and species present during winemaking, *Saccharomyces* possess a range of singular characteristics that are not found in other genera, such as the high capacity to ferment sugars, the high alcohol tolerance and the great ability to compete with other species and to colonize the wine medium [2]. The non-*Saccharomyces* yeasts are also commonly known by winemakers and wine microbiologists. This term includes many different yeast species. The current taxonomy recognizes around 149 yeasts genera and 1500 species, and more than 40 species have been isolated from grapes and grape juices [3]. *Dekkera* (anamorph form of *Brettanomyces*), *Candida* (anamorph form of *Metschnikowia*), *Cryptococcus*, *Debaryomyces*, *Hanseniaspora* (anamorph form of *Kloeckera*), *Kluyveromyces or Lachancea, Pichia*, *Rhodotorula*, *Saccharomycodes*, *Schizosaccharomyces*, *Torulaspora* and *Zygosaccharomyces* are the well-known non-*Saccharomyces* genera [4]. Generally, the non-*Saccharomyces* yeasts are commonly known as wild yeasts, because they are mostly present in grapevines, grape clusters and berry surfaces. The wild microbiota found in grapes and, therefore, in musts is affected by many external factors, such as the geographical location, the climatic conditions, the grape variety, the stage of maturity, the age of vines, the use of fungicides, the berry physical damages caused by fungi and even the presence of insects and birds [5–7]. Within a winemaking environment, the diversity of yeast species can be influenced by the population of cellar habitats, such as wall surfaces, equipment and oak barrels, among others. Thus, the cleaning and the cellar hygienic practices influence the winery microbiota affecting their diversity, composition and evolution. Nowadays, the actual hygienic practices used in the modern cellars seem to minimize the con-tamination by the resident cellar flora and, therefore, its diversity [8, 9]. In general, the non-*Saccharomyces* wine-related species have a low fermentation activity and a low SO_2 resistance [3]. However, they have the ability to colonize non-inoculated musts and to start the AF. They play an important role in the wine aroma complex-ity mainly due to their interesting enzymatic activities (proteases, β-glucosidases, esterases, pectinases and lipases) [10–12]. Many reports showed that the enzymatic activity of yeasts is conditioned by the pH, temperature, as well as the presence of inhibitors (sugars and ethanol) [13]. It seems that approximately 80% of the wild yeasts possesses one or more enzymes with biotechnological interest, being polyga-lacturonase the most common enzyme, followed by proteases (casein, gelatin) [14]. The β-glucosidase activity was linked to *Metschnikowia pulcherrima* species. A pro-teolytic activity was observed in *Pichia membranifaciens* and also in *Metschnikowia pulcherrima*. Furthermore, *Hanseniaspora* and *Torulaspora* genera are reported good producers of β-glucosidases, pectinases, proteases and enzymes involved in the xylan degradation [15–20]. *Lachancea thermotolerans* exhibited the activities of four carbohydrolases and three aminopeptidases. So, this strain could be an excellent candidate for improving the color and the turbidity of the red wines. Furthermore, this strain could even increase the acidity due to its ability to produce lactic acid during the AF [21, 22]. However, the secretion of each enzyme is not characteristic of a particular genus or species and depends on the strains. It is important to notice that although non-*Saccharomyces* populations were not detected at the end of the vinification, their secreted enzymes remained in the fermenting media [16].

LAB are the second important group of wine microorganisms, which are also present in grapes. The LAB of wines, musts and grapes belong to the genera *Oenococcus, Pediococcus, Lactobacillus* and *Leuconostoc* [23]. LAB can be homofermentative and producing exclusively lactic acid and CO_2 from sugars (glucose and/or fructose) or can be heterofermentative and also producing ethanol, acetic acid and CO_2. Generally, the MLF is conducted by *O. oeni*, which presents a heterofermentative metabolism. Other species of the mentioned genera, such as *P. pentosaceus* and *P. damnosus*, have a homofermentative metabolism, while *Lactobacillus casei* and *Lactobacillus plantarum* have been described as facultative heterofermentative. Other *Lactobacillus* species, such as *brevis* and *hilgardii*, are strictly heterofermentative [23, 24]. The acetic acid bacteria are considered spoilage microorganisms during winemaking. Their metabolism is strictly aerobic, and their principal property is that they can oxidize ethanol into acetic acid by the acetaldehyde pathway. Finally, the fungi found in vines, such as *Botryotinia*, *Uncinula*, *Alternaria*, *Plamapara*, *Aspergillus*, *Penicillium*, *Rhizopus*, *Oidium* and *Cladosporium*, can infect and colonize grapes prior to harvest and to be present in musts [25]. *Botryotinia fuckeliana* (or its anamorph form *Botrytis cinerea*), *Aspergillus* spp. and *Penicillium* spp. are able to produce metabolites that can delay the growth of yeasts during the fermentation. Furthermore, the fungi growth on grapes may contribute to the growth of some acetic acid bacteria on the grape surface.

3. Population dynamics

The main important microorganisms present in grapes are yeasts and in a minor proportion LAB, acetic acid bacteria and fungi. The content and diversity strongly depend on the sanitary status of grapes. Although grape musts are relatively complete in nutrients, its low pH and its high sugar content convert them in a selective media in which only a few bacteria and yeasts species can grow. The number of yeasts on the grape berry just before harvest varies from 10^3 to 10^6 cells/mL depending on the abovementioned factors [26]. The predominant wild species on the surface of grape berries are *Candida*, *Hanseniaspora*, *Hansenula*, *Metschnikowia* and *Pichia*. The *S. cerevisiae* population is very low in grapes [27], while the non-*Saccharomyces* could proliferate up to reach about 10^6–10^7 cells/mL populations, although it declines at mid-fermentation. *S. cerevisiae* species are the most alcohol-tolerant yeast and can reach populations of at least 10^7–10^8 cells/mL [26]. Thus, at the last stage of fermentation, they become predominant and complete the process. Besides, some species of *Brettanomyces*, *Kluyveromyces*, *Schizosaccharomyces*, *Torulaspora* and *Zygosaccharomyces* may also be present in wine during fermentation. Some of these species are considered spoilage microorganisms because they produce metabolites with an undesirable impact in wine [8].

Regarding LAB, the population and behavior mainly depend on the pH and the SO_2 content, and they can reach 10^2–10^4 cells/mL populations after grape crushing. In general, an increase on the pH involves higher LAB populations and diversity. At this initial fermentation stage, the four genera abovedescribed can be commonly identified, although the greatest diversity of LAB species is mainly detected during the AF. During the first days of the AF, the LAB population generally increases to a maximum of 10^4 cells/mL and then decreases until 10^2 cells/mL.

At the end of the AF, *O. oeni* is commonly the only species identified and remains in a latent phase waiting to the proper conditions to start the MLF. The MLF starts when their population achieves values around 10^6 cells/mL and the environment conditions are adequate (pH, ethanol, temperature and SO_2 content) [28]. As soon as the malic acid is completely degraded, the bacterial population begins to decline [24, 29].

4. Spontaneous and inoculated fermentations

There are a lot of different species in grapes that can participate on the wine fermentations. In general, the AF is conducted by a mixture of yeasts species [5]. The AF can be conducted spontaneously without inoculating any yeast strains or by the inoculation of the specific strains, commercial or wild. The most common worldwide practice is the use of commercial starters from *S. cerevisiae* to ensure a reproducible, predictable and controlled fermentation. The use of commercial wine yeasts can influence the natural microflora of musts and often leads to its removal. Wines produced under this practice show low variability, complexity and typicity with analytical and sensory properties often similar [1]. In contrast, the spontaneous fermentations have some problems to predict their evolution, due to the variability on the microbiota that comes from the grapes. However, wines produced under this kind of fermentation have greater complexity and present higher differentiating notes and character [30]. In the inoculated fermentations, *S. cerevisiae* is the most common active dry wine yeast (ADWY) used as starter culture since it offers a great control on the fermentation evolution. Currently, a wide commercial ADWY yeast strains and species are available for cellars.

The MLF is not always successful even if it is conducted by inoculated commercial *O. oeni* strains. Some reports showed the presence of different species in spontaneous MLF, although, as mentioned, *O. oeni* has been described as the principal species. The evolution of the MLF and the diversity species of LAB implicated in this process may modulate the composition of wine (pH, the ethanol content, etc.), the fermentation temperature, the winemaking technology used, the geographical region and also the yeast strains employed during the AF [31–35]. As in the case of yeasts, to develop a correct spontaneous MLF, a wild bacterial starter is needed, which is well adapted to the specific producing area and to the cellar conditions. LAB inoculation is recommended in modern and industrial wineries in order to control the evolution of the MLF. Fast and reliable fermentations are essential to obtain a high-quality wine [36]. However, the use of commercial starters shows some controversies because of the homogeneity and standardization of wines, limiting their organoleptic properties [37].

In summary, the use of wild yeast and LAB can be used to define the typicity of the wines of a region. Some authors stated that the microflora diversity is characteristic of a given area and could be considered its microbiological fingerprint [38, 39]. The inoculation of selected wild yeast and LAB species could help to control the development of the AF and MLF and to improve the complexity and could typify the wine of a region [1].

5. Fermentation end-products and wild microorganisms

Numerous fermentation end-products contribute to the aroma and flavor characteristics of wines, which determine their quality and final complexity. As it is known, wine is made up of thousands of aromatic compounds, and a large part of them are produced or transformed during the AF and MLF [40]. As mentioned above, these processes are carried out by wild or commercial strains. The use of wild strains allows us to obtain wines with a unique expression with representative characteristics of each variety and area. The aromatic profile of wines is determined by varietal aromas (from grapes), fermentative aromas (produced by yeast and LAB during fermentations) and post-fermentative aromas (associated to the aging period). The fermentative aromas clearly influence the final quality of wines, and the strains used during winemaking are responsible for the presence or absence of some flavors and other non-volatile metabolites [41]. Ethanol, carbon dioxide and glycerol are the main fermentative products. Ethanol is the main volatile product of yeasts metabolism, followed by diols, higher alcohols and esters. The ethanol content influences the wine viscosity and contributes on the aroma fastening. Other important metabolites derived from AF, such as pyruvic acid, participate on the formation of secondary products namely diacetyl, keto acids, succinic acid and butanediol [23]. Succinic acid and glycerol are two of the most important by-products affecting the "body" of the wine. Succinic is the main acid produced by yeasts, and its formation is strain dependent. The tartaric acid experiment slightly changes during fermentation, and the malic acid usually decreases during MLF, although the yeasts metabolism can also modify its concentration during the AF. Regarding acetic acid, this compound may reach more than 90% of the volatile acidity, and it is one of the most important by-products that negatively affect sensory profile of wine. This acid is mainly synthetized by acetic acid bacteria but also may be synthetized by yeasts and LAB.

Other volatile acids, such as propionic and hexanoic acids, are also produced by yeasts and bacteria, as a result of the fatty acid metabolic pathway [42]. Another important, but not always desirable, secondary metabolite of wine fermentation is the acetaldehyde. This compound is the product of the decarboxylation of the pyruvate during the AF. The higher alcohols represent another group of secondary products influencing the sensory profile of wines. The concentrations of higher alcohols are influenced by factors such as the yeast strains, the concentration of amino acids (the precursors of higher alcohols), ethanol concentration, fermentation temperature, pH, composition of grape must, aeration, etc. The higher alcohols are also important precursors for the ester formation; both of them are associated with pleasant aromas, although at high concentrations they can be undesirable.

LAB modulate the flavors of wines by modifying their chemical composition and, therefore, its sensory properties. LAB are responsible to maintain the result of the yeasts metabolism and to increase the complexity and microbial stability of the wine [24]. LAB decrease the wine acidity by the decarboxylation of malic acid to lactic acid, and they also contribute to the aroma by metabolizing other acids such as citric acid. The degradation of citric acid produces acetic acid and diacetyl, both of which have an important and undesirable effect on the wine flavor. Other metabolites affected by LAB metabolism, which have an impact on wine flavor, are alcohols, such as glycerol and mannitol, or carbonyls such as acetaldehyde and diacetyl. Finally, esters can also be modified for LAB species, including ethyl acetate, ethyl hexanoate, ethyl lactate and ethyl octanoate [42]. Depending on the species or even on the strains, LAB may be beneficial or detrimental to wine quality [29]. Meanwhile, acetic acid bacteria, as mentioned above, are only spoilage microorganism because they lead to the formation of such major oxidized aromas (acetaldehyde, acetic acid and ethyl acetate).

During the spontaneous AF, the development of many aromatic compounds occurs, mainly those belonging to the families of alcohols, ethyl esters, fatty acids, acetates and carbonyls. Aliphatic esters and alcohols seem to be more influenced than acids and carbonic compounds. In addition, terpenes and norisoprenoids, well-known primary aromas, can be provided by the wild yeasts during fermentation [43, 44]. The main aromatic descriptors of all of them are the fruity and floral notes, always appreciated in wines. The use of wild yeast to conduct a spontaneous AF may produce higher concentration of alcohols (1- hexanol, phenylethanol), terpenes and other aromatic compounds, such as β-phenyl acetate and γ-nonalactone, compared to wines produced by selected yeasts [45]. The selection of indigenous *S. cerevisiae* in red musts and its effect in their aromatic profile have been studied. The results showed that the produced wines had greater content of aromas and color intensity. These native yeasts synthesized higher content of linalool and citronellol, which exceeded their sensory limits [46].

The most related aromas of the inoculated MLFs are commonly associated with butter, yogurt, sulfur and toasted notes. Moreover, during spontaneous MLFs, the formation of many aromatic compounds is affected. Some studies have demonstrated the biosynthesis of the aromatic compounds produced during this kind of fermentations and its sensory repercussion. A reduction of herbaceous and vegetable aromas has been highlighted, and the appearance of fruity and floral aromas has been reported [47]. The changes produced in the aromatic composition of Tempranillo wines during spontaneous MLF by using wild LAB have been reported, showing significant increase in esters, lactones, terpenes, norisoprenoids and volatile phenols, such as vanillin and furfural [48].

6. Selection of wild yeast and lactic acid bacteria

For the selection of wild yeasts and LAB species of a specific wine region, first, it is needed to conduct a biodiversity study, knowing which species are present in grapes. After that, knowing the species at the different stages of a spontaneous fermentation, at the beginning, middle and end of fermentation, is essential. The first stage is to conduct a spontaneous fermentation. Then, isolate different colonies at each stage of the fermentation to obtain a collection of the different microorganisms implied. The second stage is to identify and typify each colony. The recovery and the molecular characterization of a high number of yeasts and LAB strains should be considered to establish a strain collection of oenological interest.

For the yeast species identification, different techniques could be applied. The restriction analysis of ribosomal gens is the simplest technique, reliable and extended [10, 49]. Nevertheless, several available techniques, such as microsatellites (SSRs), Rapid Amplification of Polymorphic DNA (RAPD-PCR), Pulsed-Field Gel Electrophoresis (PFGE) and DNA array technology, have been used to typify yeast strains. Between all these techniques, the more usual techniques for their simplicity and reproducibility are the restriction analysis of mitochondrial DNA [50] and the amplification of delta elements [51]. PCR-based methods have been already successfully used to identify LAB in different wines. To identify different LAB species, a good technique, fast and reliable, is the Restriction analysis of the amplified 16S-rDNA (ARDRA-PCR) [52, 53]. RAPD-PCR (Random Amplified Polymorphic DNA) is considered to be a suitable method to typify *O. oeni* strains in winemaking [54], such as PFGE (Pulse Field Gel Electrophoresis) of DNA digested with *Sfi*I [24].

Once the wild species and strains are identified and typified, the next step is to characterize each isolated strain, which has different genetic profile between them and between commercial yeast. Performing micro-fermentations with pure inoculations of all the strains with the specific characteristics of wine region must in order to test relevant species starter kits. With a better understanding of the different yeasts properties, the yeast selection procedure can be adapted to acquire strains that could improve the wine quality [55]. The AF and MLF performance by selected strains at winery conditions is the last step of selection.

The wild starter kit can be a single strain of *S. cerevisiae* or a mixture of *S. cerevisiae* and non-*Saccharomyces* species. The main trends in wine biotechnology is the use of different non-*Saccharomyces* species as starter cultures, such as *Torulaspora delbrueckii*, *Pichia kluyveri*, *Lachancea thermotolerans*, *Metschnikowia pulcherrima*, *Hanseniaspora uvarum*, *Schizosaccharomyces pombe*, etc. This practice combines the advantages of recovering features from traditional spontaneous fermentation, with a control of the vinification process, decreasing the risk associated with the microbial spoilage. The different species of non-*Saccharomyces* yeast starters are generally used in either sequential or simultaneous inoculation with *S. cerevisiae* [56]. Several studies have shown that the mixed inoculation starter kit with *S. cerevisiae* and non-*Saccharomyces* species can contribute positively to wine flavor. *M. pulcherrima* decreases volatile acidity [57], *H. uvarum* increases ester content in wine [58] and *Schizosaccharomyces pombe* deacidifies musts and increases the synthesis of glycerol and pyruvic acid [59]. In mixed fermentation, the interactions between the different yeasts composing the starter culture can led the stability of the final product and the analytical and aromatic profile [60].

The LAB selection as starters requires an ecological study and the characterization of useful technological and physiological features of the isolated strains in order to select the ones that are potentially more suitable for industrial applications. The selection of LAB for wine inoculation is essentially based on the survival of this strain and the consumption of malic acid. However, there are other important properties that are required to study the ability to produce biogenic amines and different enzymatic activities related to the final aroma profile. *O. oeni* is the preferred starter species because of its resistance to the alcohol, pH and SO_2 content. The ability to resistance the harsh wine conditions is strictly strain dependent. Furthermore, *O. oeni* ensures control of the time and the rate of MLF, reducing the potential for spoilage microorganisms and, finally, giving positive effects on flavor and aroma [61]. The development of the *Lactobacilli* and *Pediococci* in wine samples was linked to the decrease in wine quality [23]. González-Arenzana et al. demonstrated a high diversity *O. oeni* in spontaneous MLF and the complexity of the ecology involved [24]. They suggested a successful adaptation to winemaking conditions for some strains and also their potential utility for the selection of wild LAB starter cultures as individual or mixed strains.

The selection of microorganisms has been successfully used to improve the technological properties of different wines as well as their sensorial profiles helping in the production of wines without sulfites, reducing the levels of ethanol, increasing the glycerol content, varying the acidity of the must and realizing different aromatic components. In summary, the selection of wild yeast and LAB offers the best way to obtain different species and strains, which could improve the oenological characteristics and sensorial profile of wines, giving tools to the oenologist to direct their wine fermentation process. The exploitation of the microbial diversity that exists in the vineyards and in the cellars with the selection of wild yeast and LAB strains has been considered an interesting approach to overcome the distinctive peculiarities of wines produced in different regions [57].

7. Wild yeasts and lactic acid bacteria from viticultural Spanish regions

This section summarizes several studies carried out in VITEC (Wine Technology Center) from different grape varieties and Spanish regions. The isolation, identification and selection of wild yeasts and LAB were performed in 2016 and 2017 vintages, from grapes and spontaneous fermentations. The grape varieties studied were Verdejo from D.O. Rueda, Albariño from D.O. Rías Baixas and Tempranillo from D.O. Ribera del Duero and D.O.Q. Rioja. In all the cases, different species of

S. cerevisiae, non-*Saccharomyces* species and LAB were identified (**Tables 1** and **2**). **Table 1** shows the different non-*Saccharomyces* species found for each grape variety and region. The results showed that a great variety of yeasts species and strains present in grapes during spontaneous fermentation has been reported. Up to fourteen different strains of *S. cerevisiae* and seven species of non-*Saccharomyces* were identified in Verdejo. Seventy strains of *S. cerevisiae* and nine species of non-*Saccharomyces* were identified in Albariño, only at 2017. Seventy-eight strains of *S. cerevisiae* and ten non-*Saccharomyces* species were identified from Tempranillo in both regions. The non-*Saccharomyces* species were isolated in order to be inoculated together with a selected *S. cerevisiae* strain in mixed cultures. As mentioned, some of the used species are described as interesting wild yeasts, since they are able to led desirable compounds and metabolites to improve the wine quality (*Torulaspora delbrueckii*, *Pichia kluyveri*, *Lachancea thermotolerans*, *Candida*/*Metschnikowia pulcherrima* and *Hanseniaspora* species). It has been reported that *T. delbrueckii* can produce lower levels of volatile acidity than *S. cerevisiae*. *M. pulcherrima* can produce high concentrations of esters, especially ethyl octanoate; *Starmerella bacillaris* can produce high levels of glycerol and *Hanseniaspora* can improve the aromatic composition [30].

In order to study the influence of fermentation mixtures from wild selected yeasts on the wine properties, several studies were carried out in VITEC. The behavior of all yeast strains were studied, conducting fermentations at laboratory scale and at semi-industrial scale, in pure (*S. cerevisiae*) and mixed inoculations (*S. cerevisiae* and non-*Saccharomyces*). In the case of pure inoculations, significant differences were obtained in all the analyzed parameters (alcoholic degree, volatile acidity, total acidity, sulfur dioxide, glycerol and malic acid), except in the lactic acid content (data not shown). In these studies, firstly, the non-*Saccharomyces* species were inoculated and later the *S. cerevisiae* strains. In these mixed inoculations, the differences obtained depended on the time of the inoculation of the *S. cerevisiae* strain. As later the inoculation of *S. cerevisiae* is done, more differences were obtained. The inoculation time

Non-*Saccharomyces* species	Verdejo Rueda	Albariño Rías Baixas	Tempranillo R. del Duero	Tempranillo Rioja
Metschnikowia pulcherrima	√	√		√
Hanseniaspora vineae			√	√
Torulaspora delbrueckii	√	√	√	
Lanchacea thermotolerans			√	√
Hanseniaspora guillermondii	√	√		
Issatchenkia orientalis	√			
Pichia kluyveri	√			
Hanseniaspora uvarum	√	√	√	√
Aureobasidium pullulans			√	√
Rhodotorula glutinis		√		
Cryptococcus flavescens		√		
Cryptococcus magnus		√		
Starmerella bacillaris		√		
Pichia membranifaciens		√		

Table 1.
Identification of non-Saccharomyces species at different grape varieties and Spanish regions.

LAB species	Tempranillo Ribera del Duero	Tempranillo Rioja
Lactobacillus delbrueckii	√	
Lactobacillus helveticus	√	√
Lactobacillus hilgardii	√	√
Lactobacillus fermentum	√	
Lactobacillus pentosus	√	
Lactobacillus collinoides		√
Pediococcus acidilacticii		√
Oenococcus oeni	√	√

Table 2.
Identification of LAB species in Tempranillo grapes.

affected the basic oenological parameters and the aromatic fermentative compounds, including higher alcohols, esters, acetates and acids.

Concerning LAB, the highest diversity was found at the beginning of the AF. Up to eight different wild LAB species and fourteen *O. oeni* strains were identified. The fermentative characteristics of different *O. oeni* strains were studied. The results showed that some of these strains were able to conduct MLFs when the alcoholic degree did not exceed 14.5 vol., both in low and high pH wines (pH ranged from 3.3 to 4).

8. Conclusions

Wild yeasts and lactic acid bacteria are interesting microorganisms that contribute to differentiate the wine character. The suitable use of numerous wild species and strains during winemaking favors the improvement of the complexity and the organoleptic properties of wines. The production of wines by spontaneous or inoculated fermentations using selected wild microorganisms is a remarkable practice for wineries. Further studies should be done in order to deep into the knowledge of the wild microflora of grapes and wines to better understand their behavior and importance. Even more, some drastic physical and chemical winemaking techniques, increasingly used in wineries, could be replaced taking advantage of the biological properties of these microorganisms. Above all, wild yeast and lactic acid bacteria may help to produce modern and new wine styles in a climate change viticultural environment.

Acknowledgements

We thank MINECO and CDTI for their financial support through the projects MICROSEL (RTC-2016-5559-2) and GLOBALVITI (CIEN Program Ref.IDI-20160746), respectively. Thanks bodegas Matarromera S.L. (Valbuena de Duero, Valladolid, Spain) and Martín Codax SA (Cambados, Pontevedra, Spain) for supplying samples.

Conflict of interest

We have no conflict of interest to declare.

Author details

Imma Andorrà, Gemma Miró, Noelia Espligares, Ana Maria Mislata, Miquel Puxeu and Raúl Ferrer-Gallego*
VITEC, Wine Technology Center, Tarragona, Spain

*Address all correspondence to: raul.ferrer@vitec.wine

References

[1] Fleet GH. Wine yeasts for the future. FEMS Yeast Research. 2008;**8**(7):979-995. DOI: 10.1111/j.1567-1364.2008.00427.x

[2] Barrio E, Gonzalez SS, Arias A, Belloch C, Querol A. Yeast in Food Beverages. Berlin, Heidelberg: Springer Verlag; 2006

[3] Ciani M, Comitini F, Mannazzu I, Domizio P. Controlled mixed culture fermentation: A new perspective on the use of non-Saccharomyces yeasts in winemaking. Fems Yeast Research. 2010;**10**(2):123-133. DOI: 10.1111/j.1567-1364.2009.00579.x

[4] Pretorius IS, van der Westhuizen TJ, Augustyn OPH. Yeast biodiversity in vineyards and wineries and its importance to the South African wine industry. A review. South African Journal of Enology and Viticulture. 2017;**20**(2):10. DOI: 10.21548/20-2-2234

[5] Jolly NP, Augustyn OPH, Pretorius IS. The occurrence of non-*Saccharomyces cerevisiae* yeast species over three vintages in four vineyards and grape musts from four production regions of the Western Cape, South Africa. South African Journal of Enology an Viticulture. 2017;**24**(2):8. DOI: 10.21548/24-2-2640

[6] Martini A, Ciani M, Scorzetti G. Direct enumeration and isolation of wine yeasts from grape surfaces. American Journal of Enology and Viticulture. 1996;**47**(4):435-440

[7] Barata A, Seborro F, Belloch C, Malfeito-Ferreira M, Loureiro V. Ascomycetous yeast species recovered from grapes damaged by honeydew and sour rot. Journal of Applied Microbiology. 2008;**104**(4):1182-1191. DOI: 10.1111/j.1365-2672.2007.03631.x

[8] Pretorius IS. Tailoring wine yeast for the new millennium: Novel approaches to the ancient art of winemaking. Yeast. 2000;**16**(8):675-729. DOI: 10.1002/1097-0061(20000615)16:8<675::AID-YEA585>3.0.CO;2-B

[9] Rementeria A, Rodriguez JA, Cadaval A, Amenabar R, Muguruza JR, Hernando FL, et al. Yeast associated with spontaneous fermentations of white wines from the "Txakoli de Bizkaia" region (Basque Country, North Spain). International Journal of Food Microbiology. 2003;**86**(1-2):201-207. DOI: 10.1016/s0168-1605(03)00289-7

[10] Esteve-Zarzoso B, Belloch C, Uruburu F, Querol A. Identification of yeasts by RFLP analysis of the 5.8S rRNA gene and the two ribosomal internal transcribed spacers. International Journal of Systematic Bacteriology. 1999;**49**:329-337. DOI: 10.1099/00207713-49-1-329

[11] Santamaría P, Garijo P, López R, Tenorio C, Rosa Gutiérrez A. Analysis of yeast population during spontaneous alcoholic fermentation: Effect of the age of the cellar and the practice of inoculation. International Journal of Food Microbiology. 2005;**103**(1):49-56. DOI: 10.1016/j.ijfoodmicro.2004.11.024

[12] Mercado L, Dalcero A, Masuelli R, Combina M. Diversity of Saccharomyces strains on grapes and winery surfaces: Analysis of their contribution to fermentative flora of Malbec wine from Mendoza (Argentina) during two consecutive years. Food Microbiology. 2007;**24**(4):403-412. DOI: 10.1016/j.fm.2006.06.005

[13] Maturano YP, Rodríguez Assaf LA, Toro ME, Nally MC, Vallejo M, Castellanos de Figueroa LI, et al. Multi-enzyme production by pure and

mixed cultures of Saccharomyces and non-Saccharomyces yeasts during wine fermentation. International Journal of Food Microbiology. 2012;**155**(1):43-50. DOI: 10.1016/j.ijfoodmicro.2012.01.015

[14] Fernández M, Úbeda JF, Briones AI. Typing of non-Saccharomyces yeasts with enzymatic activities of interest in wine-making. International Journal of Food Microbiology. 2000;**59**(1):29-36. DOI: 10.1016/S0168-1605(00)00283-X

[15] Charoenchai C, Fleet GH, Henschke PA, Todd BENT. Screening of non-Saccharomyces wine yeasts for the presence of extracellular hydrolytic enzymes. Australian Journal of Grape and Wine Research. 1997;**3**(1):2-8. DOI: 10.1111/j.1755-0238.1997.tb00109.x

[16] Ganga MA, Martínez C. Effect of wine yeast monoculture practice on the biodiversity of non-Saccharomyces yeasts. Journal of Applied Microbiology. 2004;**96**(1):76-83. DOI: 10.1046/j.1365-2672.2003.02080.x

[17] Manzanares P, Ramón D, Querol A. Screening of non-Saccharomyces wine yeasts for the production of beta-D-xylosidase activity. International Journal of Food Microbiology. 1999;**46**(2):105-112. DOI: 10.1016/s0168-1605(98)00186-x

[18] Pérez G, Fariña L, Barquet M, Boido E, Gaggero C, Dellacassa E, et al. A quick screening method to identify β-glucosidase activity in native wine yeast strains: Application of esculin glycerol agar (EGA) medium. World Journal of Microbiology and Biotechnology. 2011;**27**(1):47-55. DOI: 10.1007/s11274-010-0425-4

[19] Romo-Sánchez S, Alves-Baffi M, Arévalo-Villena M, Úbeda-Iranzo J, Briones-Pérez A. Yeast biodiversity from oleic ecosystems: Study of their biotechnological properties. Food Microbiology. 2010;**27**(4):487-492. DOI: 10.1016/j.fm.2009.12.009

[20] Masoud W, Jespersen L. Pectin degrading enzymes in yeasts involved in fermentation of Coffea arabica in East Africa. International Journal of Food Microbiology. 2006;**110**(3):291-296. DOI: 10.1016/j.ijfoodmicro.2006.04.030

[21] Escribano R, González-Arenzana L, Garijo P, Berlanas C, López-Alfaro I, López R, et al. Screening of enzymatic activities within different enological non-Saccharomyces yeasts. Journal of Food Science and Technology. 2017;**54**(6):1555-1564. DOI: 10.1007/s13197-017-2587-7

[22] Gobbi M, Comitini F, Domizio P, Romani C, Lencioni L, Mannazzu I, et al. Lachancea thermotolerans and Saccharomyces cerevisiae in simultaneous and sequential co-fermentation: A strategy to enhance acidity and improve the overall quality of wine. Food Microbiology. 2013;**33**(2):271-281. DOI: 10.1016/j.fm.2012.10.004

[23] Ribéreau-Gayon P, Dubourdieu D, Donèche B, Lonvaud A. Handbook of Enology, Volume 1: The Microbiology of Wine and Vinifications. 2nd ed. Chichester, West Sussex, England: John Wiley & Sons Ltd; 2006

[24] Gonzalez-Arenzana L, Lopez R, Santamaria P, Tenorio C, Lopez-Alfaro I. Dynamics of indigenous lactic acid bacteria populations in wine fermentations from La Rioja (Spain) during three vintages. Microbial Ecology. 2012;**63**(1):12-19. DOI: 10.1007/s00248-011-9911-y

[25] Fleet GH. Wine. In: Food Microbiology Fundamentals and Frontiers. 2nd ed. Washington, USA: ASM Press; 2001

[26] Romano P, Capece A, Jespersen L. Taxonomic and ecological diversity of food and beverage yeasts. In: Querol A, Fleet G, editors. Yeasts in Food and

Beverages. Berlin, Heidelberg: Springer Berlin Heidelberg; 2006. pp. 13-53

[27] Torija MJ, Rozes N, Poblet M, Guillamon JM, Mas A. Yeast population dynamics in spontaneous fermentations: Comparison between two different wine-producing areas over a period of three years. Antonie van Leeuwenhoek International Journal of General and Molecular Microbiology. 2001;**79**(3-4):345-352. DOI: 10.1023/a:1012027718701

[28] Renouf V. In: Lavoisier TD, editor. La Fermentation Malolactique dans les Vins. Mécanismes et Applications Pratiques. Paris: EMD, Lassay-les-Château; 2013

[29] Lonvaud-Funel A. Lactic acid bacteria in the quality improvement and depreciation of wine. Antonie Van Leeuwenhoek. 1999;**76**(1-4):317-331

[30] Jolly NP, Varela C, Pretorius IS. Not your ordinary yeast: Non-Saccharomyces yeasts in wine production uncovered. FEMS Yeast Research. 2014;**14**(2):215-237. DOI: 10.1111/1567-1364.12111

[31] Andorra I, Landi S, Mas A, Guillamon JM, Esteve-Zarzoso B. Effect of oenological practices on microbial populations using culture-independent techniques. Food Microbiology. 2008;**25**(7):849-856. DOI: 10.1016/j.fm.2008.05.005

[32] Guerrini S, Bastianini A, Blaiotta G, Granchi L, Moschetti G, Coppola S, et al. Phenotypic and genotypic characterization of Oenococcus oeni strains isolated from Italian wines. International Journal of Food Microbiology. 2003;**83**(1):1-14. DOI: 10.1016/s0168-1605(02)00323-9

[33] Ruiz P, Izquierdo PM, Sesena S, Palop ML. Analysis of lactic acid bacteria populations during spontaneous malolactic fermentation of Tempranillo wines at five wineries during two consecutive vintages. Food Control. 2010;**21**(1):70-75. DOI: 10.1016/j.foodcont.2009.04.002

[34] Robinson HA, Pinharanda A, Bensasson D. Summer temperature can predict the distribution of wild yeast populations. Ecology and Evolution. 2016;**6**(4):1236-1250. DOI: 10.1002/ece3.1919

[35] Robinson AL, Boss PK, Heymann H, Solomon PS, Trengove RD. Influence of yeast strain, canopy management, and site on the volatile composition and sensory attributes of cabernet sauvignon wines from Western Australia. Journal of Agricultural and Food Chemistry. 2011;**59**(7):3273-3284. DOI: 10.1021/jf104324d

[36] Di Maro E, Ercolini D, Coppola S. Yeast dynamics during spontaneous wine fermentation of the Catalanesca grape. International Journal of Food Microbiology. 2007;**117**(2):201-210. DOI: 10.1016/j.pestbp.2007.04.007

[37] Rainieri S, Pretorius IS. Selection and improvement of wine yeast. Annals of Microbiology. 2000;**50**(1):15-31. http://hdl.handle.net/10019.1/11880

[38] Bokulich NA, Thorngate JH, Richardson PM, Mills DA. Microbial biogeography of wine grapes is conditioned by cultivar, vintage, and climate. Proceedings of the National Academy of Sciences of the United States of America. 2014;**111**(1):E139-EE48. DOI: 10.1073/pnas.1317377110

[39] Mas A, Padilla B, Esteve-Zarzoso B, Beltran G, Reguant C, Bordons A. Taking advantage of natural biodiversity for wine making: The WILDWINE project. In: Menghini S, Pfoestl E, Marinelli A, editors. Florence 'Sustainability of Well-Being International Forum', 2015: Food for Sustainability and Not Just Food,

Florenceswif 2015. Agriculture and Agricultural Science Procedia. 82016. pp. 4-9

[40] Gammacurta M, Marchand S, Albertin W, Moine V, de Revel G. Impact of yeast strain on ester levels and fruity aroma persistence during aging of Bordeaux red wines. Journal of Agricultural and Food Chemistry. 2014;**62**(23):5378-5389. DOI: 10.1021/jf500707e

[41] Devi A, Archana KM, Bhavya PK, Anu-Appaiah KA. Non-anthocyanin polyphenolic transformation by native yeast and bacteria co-inoculation strategy during vinification. Journal of the Science of Food and Agriculture. 2018;**98**(3):1162-1170. DOI: 10.1002/jsfa.8567

[42] Swiegers JH, Bartowsky EJ, Henschke PA, Pretorius IS. Yeast and bacterial modulation of wine aroma and flavour. Australian Journal of Grape and Wine Research. 2005;**11**(2):139-173. DOI: 10.1111/j.1755-0238.2005.tb00285.x

[43] Robinson AL, Boss PK, Solomon PS, Trengove RD, Heymann H, Ebeler SE. Origins of grape and wine aroma. Part 1. Chemical components and viticultural impacts. American Journal of Enology and Viticulture. 2014;**65**(1):1-24. DOI: 10.5344/ajev.2013.12070

[44] Robinson AL, Boss PK, Solomon PS, Trengove RD, Heymann H, Ebeler SE. Origins of grape and wine aroma. Part 2. Chemical and sensory analysis. American Journal of Enology and Viticulture. 2014;**65**(1):25-42. DOI: 10.5344/ajev.2013.13106

[45] Synos K, Reynolds AG, Bowen AJ. Effect of yeast strain on aroma compounds in cabernet franc icewines. LWT - Food Science and Technology. 2015;**64**(1):227-235. DOI: 10.1016/j.lwt.2015.05.044

[46] Masssera A, Assof M, Sturm ME, Sari S, Jofré V, Cordero-Otero R, et al. Selection of indigenous *Saccharomyces cerevisiae* strains to ferment red musts at low temperature. Annals of Microbiology. 2012;**62**:367-380

[47] Antalick G, Perello M-C, de Revel G. Characterization of fruity aroma modifications in red wines during malolactic fermentation. Journal of Agricultural and Food Chemistry. 2012;**60**(50):12371-12383. DOI: 10.1021/jf303238n

[48] Izquierdo Cañas PM, García Romero E, Gómez Alonso S, Palop Herreros MLL. Changes in the aromatic composition of Tempranillo wines during spontaneous malolactic fermentation. Journal of Food Composition and Analysis. 2008;**21**(8):724-730. DOI: 10.1016/j.jfca.2007.12.005

[49] Guillamón JM, Sabaté J, Barrio E, Cano J, Querol A. Rapid identification of wine yeast species based on RFLP analysis of the ribosomal internal transcribed spacer (ITS) region. Archives of Microbiology. 1998;**169**(5):387-392. DOI: 10.1007/s002030050587

[50] Querol A, Barrio E, Huerta T, Ramón D. Molecular monitoring of wine fermentations conducted by active dry yeast strains. Applied and Environmental Microbiology. 1992;**58**(9):2948-2953

[51] Legras J-L, Karst F. Optimisation of interdelta analysis for Saccharomyces cerevisiae strain characterisation. FEMS Microbiology Letters. 2003;**221**(2):249-255. DOI: 10.1016/S0378-1097(03)00205-2

[52] Cappello MS, Stefani D, Grieco F, Logrieco A, Zapparoli G. Genotyping by amplified fragment length polymorphism and malate metabolism performances of indigenous Oenococcus

oeni strains isolated from Primitivo wine. International Journal of Food Microbiology. 2008;**127**(3):241-245. DOI: 10.1016/j.ijfoodmicro.2008.07.009

[53] Rodas AM, Ferrer S, Pardo I. 16S-ARDRA, a tool for identification of lactic acid bacteria isolated from grape must and wine. Systematic and Applied Microbiology. 2003;**26**(3):412-422. DOI: 10.1078/072320203322497446

[54] Araque MI, Bordons A, Reguant C. A multiplex PCR method for simultaneous species identification and strain typification of Oenococcus oeni. World Journal of Microbiology and Biotechnology. 2009;**25**(1):15-18. DOI: 10.1007/s11274-008-9854-8

[55] Suarez-Lepe JA, Morata A. New trends in yeast selection for winemaking. Trends in Food Science and Technology. 2012;**23**(1):39-50. DOI: 10.1016/j.tifs.2011.08.005

[56] Tronchoni J, Curiel JA, Morales P, Torres-Perez R, Gonzalez R. Early transcriptional response to biotic stress in mixed starter fermentations involving Saccharomyces cerevisiae and Torulaspora delbrueckii. International Journal of Food Microbiology. 2017;**241**:60-68. DOI: 10.1016/j.ijfoodmicro.2016.10.017

[57] Barbosa C, Lage P, Esteves M, Chambel L, Mendes-Faia A, Mendes-Ferreira A. Molecular and phenotypic characterization of Metschnikowia pulcherrima strains from Douro wine region. Fermentation. 2018;**4**(1):8

[58] Andorra I, Berradre M, Rozes N, Mas A, Guillamon JM, Esteve-Zarzoso B. Effect of pure and mixed cultures of the main wine yeast species on grape must fermentations. European Food Research and Technology. 2010;**231**(2):215-224. DOI: 10.1007/s00217-010-1272-0

[59] Benito S, Palomero F, Calderon F, Palmero D, Suarez-Lepe JA. Selection of appropriate Schizosaccharomyces strains for winemaking. Food Microbiology. 2014;**42**:218-224. DOI: 10.1016/j.fm.2014.03.014

[60] Ciani M, Capece A, Comitini F, Canonico L, Siesto G, Romano P. Yeast interactions in inoculated wine fermentation. Frontiers in Microbiology. 2016;7:555. DOI: 10.3389/fmicb.2016.00555

[61] Solieri L, Genova F, De Paola M, Giudici P. Characterization and technological properties of Oenococcus oeni strains from wine spontaneous malolactic fermentations: A framework for selection of new starter cultures. Journal of Applied Microbiology. 2010;**108**(1):285-298. DOI: 10.1111/j.1365-2672.2009.04428.x

Chapter 5

Biotechnological Applications of Nonconventional Yeasts

Camila de Souza Varize, Renata Maria Christofoleti-Furlan, Elisangela de Souza Miranda Muynarsk, Gilberto Vinícius de Melo Pereira, Lucas Dantas Lopes and Luiz Carlos Basso

Abstract

Yeasts not belonging to species of the *Saccharomyces* genus, called nonconventional yeasts, have gained prominence recently in the biotechnological scenario. For many years, they have been generally characterized as undesirable contaminants in fermentative processes. However, several studies pointed them as useful for many biotechnological applications. This chapter will cover some of these applications, highlighting the most widely employed nonconventional yeasts. The use of non-*Saccharomyces* strains in (I) xylose fermentation for the production of ethanol and xylitol, (II) brewing industry, (III) improvement of coffee and cocoa fermentation, and (IV) plant growth promotion will be presented.

Keywords: nonconventional yeasts, xylose fermentation, brewing industry, coffee/cocoa fermentation, plant growth promotion

1. Introduction

Yeasts have been extensively exploited by humanity for the production of bread, alcoholic beverages, bioethanol, biomass (as human or animal protein supplement), and glycerol [1–4]. They are suitable models for studies of molecular genetics, biotechnology, evolutionary biology, genomics, and eukaryotic cell biology due to their ease of culture, simple and relatively fast life cycles, and small genomes [5]. The most known species of yeasts belong to the subphylum Saccharomycotina, including *Saccharomyces cerevisiae* (eukaryotic model system), *Candida albicans* (common human commensal and opportunistic pathogen), and over 1000 other species. These eukaryotic single-celled microorganisms are found in every biome and continent and are more genetically diverse than chordates or angiosperms [5].

The different applications of yeasts represent one of the oldest uses of biotechnology by mankind. Although *S. cerevisiae* is the most domesticated and widely used industrial yeast, many other yeast species that evolved over half-a-billion years have been overshadowed, but could also show a high biotechnological potential [5–7]. A variety of other yeast genera and species than *Saccharomyces*—called nonconventional yeasts—may support experimental studies and favor the biotechnological generation of value-added products [8, 9].

The wide variety of nonconventional yeasts has gained attention for numerous applications in the areas of biocatalysis (pharmaceuticals, chemical intermediates, and biotransformations), biofuels, alcoholic beverages (enhancement of desirable flavors), fundamental biological research (molecular and cellular biology, genomics, functional genomics, pathway engineering, and system biology mechanisms), biomedical research (drug discovery, drug resistance and metabolism, and elucidation of disease mechanism), biocontrol (crop protection, food and feed safety, and probiotics), environmental biotechnology (bioremediation and pollutant degradation), and heterologous protein production (protein pharmaceuticals, enzymes, hormones, vaccines, and toxins) [10–14].

In this chapter, we mined the literature in order to present some applications of nonconventional yeasts. First, a metabolism not present in *S. cerevisiae*, the fermentation of the pentose sugar xylose, is addressed whose process can generate both ethanol and xylitol as the final products. The metabolic pathway, the main nonconventional yeast species able to perform this activity, and the challenges of the process are discussed. Then, the potential of nonconventional yeasts for the production of new flavors and aroma attributes in the production of craft beer, coffee, and chocolate is described. The chapter is finished with a review regarding an alternative biotechnological application of yeasts, the use of nonconventional strains able to perform many activities associated with plant growth promotion.

2. Some applications of nonconventional yeasts

2.1 Xylose fermentation

The world energy scenario urgently needs alternative sources for replacing fossil-based fuels, mainly because of the damage that they cause to the environment [15]. Petroleum-based fuels are the most widely used, a scenario that involves high costs and climate concerns [16, 17]. The burning of fuels such as gasoline and diesel contributes to the release of most of the gases causing the greenhouse effect [17, 18]. For these reasons, biofuels are attractive alternatives to the finite fossil fuels [19]. Bioethanol is a promising example of clean and renewable energy source. It is the most widely used biofuel worldwide, both in pure form or as a gasoline additive [20].

Brazil is the world's second largest ethanol producer, whereas USA is the leader using corn starch as the fermenting substrate [21]. However, the main raw materials used for obtaining fermentable substrates, *i.e.* corn, sugarcane, and sugar beet, also show food destinations that raise a recurrent discussion about new alternatives for ethanol production [22]. In addition, the conventional production of biofuels faces several obstacles to achieve the desired levels, encouraging the use of advanced technologies, such as ethanol produced from lignocellulosic biomass, also known as second-generation ethanol [23].

Lignocellulose has a great biotechnological value and comprises most part of the plant dry weight, composed of 35–50% of cellulose, 20–35% of hemicellulose, and 10–25% of lignin. It is the largest source of renewable organic material, highly generated through agricultural and forestry practices [24, 25]. The polysaccharide components of the lignocellulosic biomass (cellulose and hemicellulose) can be processed through a hydrolysis reaction to release sugar monomers, such as hexoses and pentoses (especially glucose and xylose, respectively) that can be used as substrates in fermentation processes [26, 27]. Xylose has a high biotechnological potential; it is the most abundant sugar of the biosphere after glucose. D-xylose can be used by nonconventional yeasts for the bioconversion to ethanol or xylitol [28, 29], while *Saccharomyces cerevisiae*—the most widely employed yeast species in fermentative processes—is not able to metabolize it [30–32]. In this context, exploring the biodiversity of yeast strains not belonging to *Saccharomyces cerevisiae* species for xylose fermentation is of fundamental importance.

Xylitol has a sweetening power similar to sucrose and is found in nature, fruits, and vegetables. It is effective in sucrose substitution, since its metabolism is independent of insulin, which allows its utilization in the treatment of diabetes [33–36]. Due to its physical and chemical properties, xylitol is a compound of high added value, attracting high interest of the pharmaceutical, food, and dentifrice industries. Moreover, its proven efficiency in reducing the incidence of tooth decay promoted application in the oral health field [37–39]. The concentration of xylitol in plants is relatively low; thus, it is not economically feasible to extract it. On the other hand, bacteria, filamentous fungi, and non-*Saccharomyces* yeast species are microorganisms capable of performing an efficient bioconversion of D-xylose to xylitol. Yeasts belonging to the genus *Candida* are especially known for the capacity to perform this bioconversion. *C. guilliermondii* and *C. maltosa* are species that have been identified with high rates of D-xylose consumption and xylitol production in the fermentation under microaerophilic conditions [40, 41].

The discovery of D-xylose-fermenting yeasts began in the 1980s [42], and since this decade, we can list some species of nonconventional yeasts studied for ethanol production: *Pachysolen tannophilus* [43], *Kluyveromyces cellobiovorus* [44], *Scheffersomyces* (*Candida*) *shehatae* [45], and *Scheffersomyces* (*Pichia*) *stipitis* [45–47]. Most recently, *Spathaspora arborariae* [48, 49], *Sp. passalidarum* [50–53], and *Sp. piracicabensis* are other species described as able to perform this activity [54]. *Spathaspora passalidarum*, *Sp. arborariae*, *Sp. piracicabensis*, *Sp. gorwiae*, *and Sp. hagerdaliae* produce ethanol mostly from D-xylose, while the remaining species within this clade are considered xylitol producers. Among the set of *Spathaspora* species able to ferment D-xylose, *Sp. passalidarum* is the highest ethanol producer under oxygen-limited or anaerobic conditions, showing rapid D-xylose consumption and also the ability to ferment glucose, xylose, and cellobiose simultaneously. *Sp. passalidarum* is a potential candidate for use in the fermentation of sugars from lignocellulosic biomass [55].

Many other *Candida* species are also reported as capable of fermenting xylose for ethanol and/or xylitol bioconversion: *C. tenuis* (*Yamadazyma tenuis*), *C. tropicalis*, *C. utilis* (*Cyberlindnera jadinii*), *C. blankii*, *C. friedrichii*, *C. solani*, and *C. parapsilosis*. Also described as xylose fermenters are species of the genera *Debaryomyces*, *Brettanomyces*, *Clavispora*, and *Schizosaccharomyces* [56–58].

The hydrolysis reaction of the lignocellulose biomass is conducted first through a pretreatment that can be mechanical, chemical, or heat-based. It is performed in order to reduce the amount of lignin and enable the following enzymatic hydrolysis of the polysaccharides [59]. Although there are many studies with particular species able to ferment D-xylose, the conversion of this pentose into ethanol still faces a high number of challenges, such as (I) metabolic repression due to a fermentation involving a mix of pentose and hexose sugars present in hydrolyzed substrate, (II) the presence of toxic substances generated by the pretreatment and hydrolysis reaction (furfural and acetic acid), (III) the unbalance between coenzymes required by the enzymes associated to the early stages of xylose metabolism, and (IV) the need of an oxygen supply for ethanol production [32]. Therefore, ethanol production from D-xylose has not yet reached commercial levels, which requires deeper studies aiming to achieve an appropriate conversion process [60]. The exploitation of yeasts for D-xylose fermentation is also limited by the low tolerance of cells to ethanol, slow fermentation rates, and also the difficulty in controlling the rate of oxygen supply at an optimum level during fermentation. The combined presence of sugars (hexose and pentose) present in the hydrolysate also introduces difficulties as mentioned above [61], because hexoses can inhibit D-xylose metabolism by repression and inactivation of the D-xylose transport systems or catabolic enzymes [62].

Throughout the biosphere, microbial diversity is poorly known and represents a huge potential source for the discovery of new species [63, 64]. This untapped biodiversity probably contains species able to ferment D-xylose and other sugars efficiently. Bioprospection and identification of new yeasts capable of fermenting sugars from lignocellulosic biomass are of particular interest for the development of technologies aiming to produce biofuels in a useful and viable way. D-xylose fermenting yeasts have been isolated for example from the gut of wood-boring insects such as passalid beetles (*S. stipitis, S. shehatae, Sp. passalidarum, C. jeffriesii,* and *Sp. allomyrina*) [51, 65, 66], rotting wood (*Sp. arborariae* and *Sp. piracicabensis*) [50, 54], mushrooms, bromeliads (*S. shehatae*) [67, 68], larval gut of the silkworm (*Blastobotrys bombycis*) [69], and peat in a tropical swamp forest in Surat Thani province of Thailand (*C. kantuleensis*) [70]. The prospection of species in Brazilian ecosystems has focused mainly on Atlantic Rainforest, and other few studies have been conducted on Cerrado ecosystem and Amazonian Forest sites [71]. The draft or complete genomes of the D-xylose fermenting yeasts *S. stipitis*, *Sp. arborariae*, and *Sp. xylofermentans* were already sequenced and have been studied accurately. The genes involved in the mechanisms of regulation of xylose metabolism are very important for engineering xylose metabolism in *S. cerevisiae* [72–74].

The uptake of D-xylose by yeast cells occurs through membrane-carrying proteins. D-xylose transport occurs by a facilitated diffusion mechanism; thus, the only driving force is the sugar gradient. It also occurs by an active transport system (co-transport of H^+ and sugar) [32, 75]. The metabolism of D-xylose in yeast occurs according to the descriptive scheme of **Figure 1** [29, 42, 61, 76, 77]:

1. D-xylose is initially transported into the cell;

2. With the presence of coenzymes NADH and NADPH, the enzyme xylose reductase (XR) converts xylose to xylitol, releasing NAD^+ and $NADP^+$, respectively;

3. The xylitol formed can be either excreted in the medium or oxidized to xylulose by the enzyme xylitol dehydrogenase (XDH) in the strict presence of the NAD^+ coenzyme, releasing NADH;

4. The produced xylulose is phosphorylated by the enzyme xylulokinase (XK) and forms xylulose-5-phosphate;

5. Xylulose-5-phosphate is metabolized by pentose phosphate pathway (PPP);

6. The pentose phosphate pathway (PPP) has two phases: the oxidative phase and the nonoxidative phase (regeneration phase);

7. Metabolites resulting from the pentose phosphate pathway (fructose-6P and glyceraldehyde-3P) are metabolized in glycolysis (Embden-Meyerhof route) and converted to pyruvate;

8. Pyruvate can be oxidized by the Krebs cycle and recovers the coenzymes through the respiratory chain, or it can also be fermented into ethanol by the action of pyruvate decarboxylase and alcohol dehydrogenase enzymes (in this process NADH is reoxidized as a result of glyceraldehyde-3P oxidation).

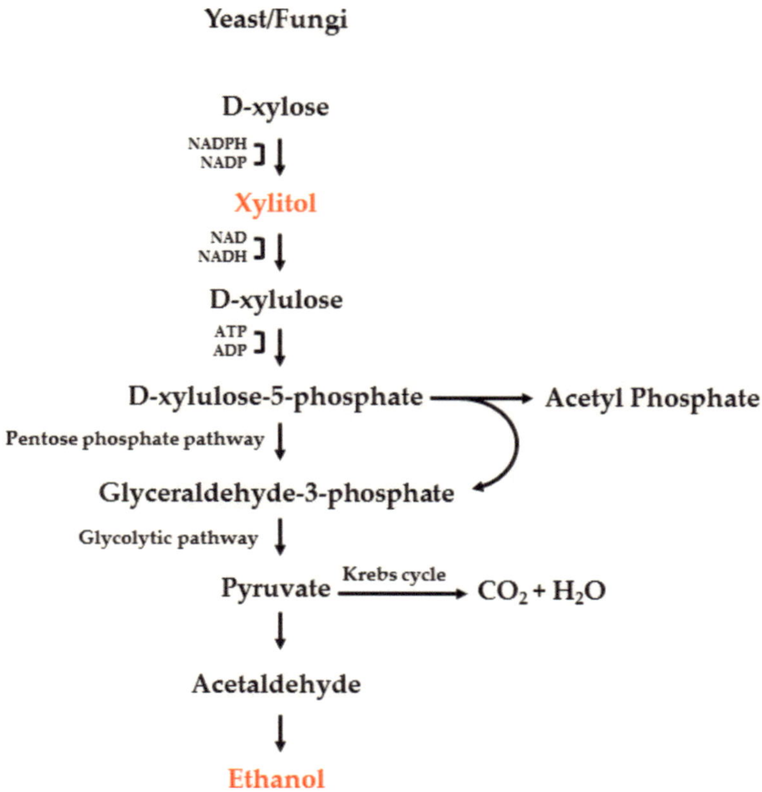

Figure 1.
Schematic diagram of D-xylose metabolism.

Understanding xylose metabolism is important for obtaining high yield fermentation. In some yeast strains, the enzyme xylose reductase (XR) is only dependent on the NADPH coenzyme, releasing $NADP^+$. In others, the XR enzyme can use both coenzymes (NADPH and NADH), releasing $NADP^+$ and NAD^+, respectively. In the following step, xylitol dehydrogenase (XDH) is strictly dependent on the NAD^+ coenzyme, causing the unbalance of coenzymes, which limits the fermentation process of D-xylose to ethanol, since this specific dependence can cause xylitol accumulation [78].

The coenzymes used by the main enzymes involved, xylose reductase (XR) and xylitol dehydrogenase (XDH), proceed with even more unbalance of coenzymes under anaerobic conditions, since the coenzyme $NADP^+$ can be reduced via fructose-6-phosphate, and the coenzyme NADH cannot be oxidized in the absence of oxygen. In this way, xylitol accumulates, and hence, ethanol production decreases [77]. Therefore, oxygenation control at the optimal level is one of the most important physiological factors. Aeration determines the division of xylose carbon flux between cell growth and bioconversion. The enzyme XR that has activity in the presence of both coenzymes can favor the production of ethanol under anaerobic conditions [79, 80].

Industrial xylitol is produced by chemical reduction of xylose. However, its biological production would be more attractive due to the low costs associated to its production and better organoleptic characteristics. The chemical production requires more energy supply, which increases the price of the product and makes it less competitive compared to other sweeteners. The biotechnological process is carried out under conditions of moderate temperature and pressure, and therefore has the lowest energy requirements. This bioconversion is highly specific, resulting in higher yields and lower costs of product separation and purification, as well as cleaner effluents [37, 81, 82]. The biotechnological production of xylitol is associated with the ability of microorganisms to synthesize the enzyme xylose reductase (XR). As mentioned above, XR catalyzes the reduction of xylose to xylitol with the participation of the NADPH or NADH. Xylitol can be either excreted from the cell or oxidized to xylulose by the enzyme xylitol dehydrogenase (XDH), whose activity requires the NAD^+ cofactor. Briefly, the production of xylitol depends on a high activity of the XR enzyme or a low activity of the enzyme XDH. The degree of activity of these enzymes is a criterion used to identify the best producers [78, 82–86].

The enzyme xylose isomerase (XI) is able to transform xylose directly into xylulose. The xylose isomerase (XI) pathway does not produce xylitol and is performed by some prokaryotes, fungi, and plants. However, such natural ability in yeasts has not yet been described. There are genetically modified strains with this enzymatic capacity [87]. Research also reports the ability of genetically modified *S. cerevisiae* strains to ferment xylose into ethanol, but these studies also raise questions about the fermentation viability [30, 32].

2.2 Beer fermentation

The most widely used yeasts for beer fermentation are of the genus *Saccharomyces*. Yeast strains belonging to the species *S. cerevisiae* and *S. pastorianus* are used for the production of the two main families of beers: ale and lager, respectively. The selection and use of *Saccharomyces* spp. (mainly *S. cerevisiae*) for controlled fermentations over time is related to several attractive traits, such as high fermentation performance, tolerance to ethanol and other stressors, production of desirable flavor and aroma compounds, and the safe use for fermented foods and beverages, *i.e.*, the absence of production of toxic metabolites [88].

Despite the widespread use of such traditional starter yeasts for brewing, the use of nonconventional yeasts, especially non-*Saccharomyces* species, has been gaining attention with the increasing demand for product innovation and diversity [89]. The growth of the craft beer segment has boosted the search for strategies to bring differentiation to the beverages, and the role of different yeasts in defining the beer traits has been exploited and gained special attention [90].

Generally, non-*Saccharomyces* yeasts present lower fermentative efficiency when compared to *Saccharomyces* spp., exhibiting reduced ethanol yield [91], and they usually have been seen as contaminant agents of the brewing process due to associated problems and negative influence on beer quality [92]. However, these yeasts may display distinct physiologic and metabolic activities, which can all contribute to secondary metabolite production, impacting on the sensorial complexity of the beer [89, 91].

The use of non-*Saccharomyces* yeast strains in the production of beers has the potential to provide distinctive flavor and aroma attributes [93]. In food and beverages, the production or enhancement of flavor compounds via (micro) biological systems is referred to as bioflavoring [94], and several non-*Saccharomyces* yeasts species have been pointed out as feasible agents to enhance, improve, and diversify the beer sensorial characteristics [95]. Besides bioflavoring, other applications have been highlighted, such as the production of low-/no-alcohol beers and light (low calorie) beers [89, 93, 95]. Non-*Saccharomyces* yeasts are commonly encountered in spontaneous and uncontrolled fermentation processes, *e.g.*, in the production of sour beers, such as Belgian lambics and American coolship ales [92]. During fermentation, a succession of autochthonous yeasts and bacteria are observed along the process, which lasts for 1–3 years in oak barrels. Among non-*Saccharomyces*, primarily *Debaryomyces* has been detected in lambic, and *Rhodotorula* in coolship ale at the first month of fermentation. Both yeasts are replaced by *Saccharomyces* spp., which dominate the main alcoholic fermentation for 3–4 months. Subsequently, the latter is gradually outcompeted by *Brettanomyces* (teleomorph *Dekkera*), mainly *B. bruxellensis*, which presents high tolerance to ethanol and remains the predominant non-*Saccharomyces* yeast until the end of fermentation (along the acidification-maturation phase) [96, 97]. During this phase, *Dekkera/Brettanomyces* contributes to a higher attenuation of the wort, due to the consumption of oligosaccharides that *Saccharomyces* is not able to metabolize, and to the production of several aroma compounds, such as caprylic and capric fatty acids and their ethyl esters, ethyl phenol, ethyl guaiacol, isovaleric acid, acetic acid, and ethyl acetate, which together characterize those particular beer styles [88, 93, 95]. Other non-*Saccharomyces* yeasts of the genera *Kluyveromyces, Torulaspora, Candida, Hanseniaspora, Pichia, Meyerozyma, Wickerhamomyces, Cryptococcus*, and *Priceomyces* have already been found in such spontaneous fermentations [92, 97], but not many of them have been evaluated to be used under controlled beer fermentations [98].

Nowadays, the most commonly used nonconventional yeast in craft and specialty beers is *Dekkera/Brettanomyces* [99]. The ability to produce a large diversity of aroma compounds, most notably phenolic compounds, ethyl esters, and (fatty) acids, has made this yeast an interesting bioflavoring agent to bring specific sensory characteristics to the beers [88, 99]. A lot of aromatic descriptors, both positive and negative, have been associated to *Dekkera/Brettanomyces* spp. ferments, including floral, fruity, citrus, spicy, clove, leather, barnyard, smoky, plastic, mousy, phenolic, medical, and/or "band-aid", which are usually called "Brett flavor" [100]. Some common beer styles in which those species can contribute to with their specific flavors include Lambic, Gueuze, and American Kettle sour (marked by sour character); Kriek, Berliner Weisse, and Brett IPA (fruity character); Saison Farmhouse ale, Belgian Trappist ale, and Old English ale (phenolic character); and Cask Brett barley wine, Old stout, and Flanders Red ale (woody character) [99].

Regarding the production of volatile phenolic compounds, the interest in some *Dekkera/Brettanomyces* spp. for use in craft and specialty beers also relies on their ability to produce ethyl phenols [99]. Their syntheses are related to hydroxycinnamic acid (ferulic, p-coumaric, and caffeic acids derived from cereal grains used for mashing) metabolization, in which two consecutive reactions catalyzed by specific enzymes are involved, phenylacrylic acid decarboxylase and vinylphenol reductase, the last one being exclusive to *Dekkera/Brettanomyces* [100, 101]. Some strains of *D/B anomala* and *D/B bruxellensis* have showed efficient conversion of ferulic acid into 4-ethyl guaiacol, making them suitable for beers in which spicy, clove-like and vanilla flavors are desired [102]. Despite the ability to metabolize hydroxycinnamic acids is strain specific, many strains suitable for brewing prefer to consume ferulic acid among other hydroxycinnamic acids [103].

Another common property of *Dekkera/Brettanomyces* is its ability to metabolize complex sugars, such as dextrins, which are not assimilable by *Saccharomyces* and account for the main residual sugars in the beer. This metabolization capacity enables its use in the production of super-attenuated and low-calorie beers [100]. These yeasts were also shown to present β-glucosidase activity, a strain dependent feature that enables the hydrolysis of glycosides present in hops, fruits, flowers, and woods, releasing more aromatic molecules, *e.g.* terpenes derived from hops [95, 99]. Furthermore, one *D. bruxellensis* expressing high β-glucosidase activity was shown to be able to produce resveratrol, a molecule with antioxidant and antiaging actions [104]. Future researches could consider such ability for the production of functional beers, which can provide health benefits for consumers.

Besides *Dekkera/Brettanomyces, Torulaspora delbrueckii* (anamorph *Candida colliculosa*) has been pointed out as a feasible agent to enhance beer bioflavor, displaying a great contribution to produce specialty beers with different flavors and aromas [89, 95, 102, 105]. These microorganisms have shown ability to produce esters and higher alcohol compounds both in pure and mixed fermentations with *Saccharomyces* spp., positively impacting on the overall analytical and sensory profile of beer [106–108]. Its co-inoculation with *S. cerevisiae* seems to raise the concentration of esters, such as both ethyl decanoate and ethyl dodecanoate as well as citronellyl acetate [105], phenyl ethyl acetate, ethyl hexanoate and ethyl octanoate [106], and ethyl acetate and isoamyl acetate [107], which can overall contribute to fruit-like flavors. Increased levels of higher alcohols, mainly amylic and isoamylic alcohol, in *S. cerevisiae/T. delbrueckii* mixed fermentations [107], and 2-phenylethanol and amyl alcohol in some *T. delbrueckii* pure fermentations [108] have also been described. The ability of some strains to augment the concentration of 4-vinyl guaiacol (clove-like descriptor), a desirable flavor in some wheat and blond beer styles, has been stood out in fermentations sequentially inoculated with *S. cerevisiae* [102] and, furthermore, pure culture of some *T. delbrueckii* has already been used to produce Hefeweizen beers (a German wheat beer style), imprinting rose, bubblegum, banana, and clove-like aromas [109]. Also, its ability to convert some monoterpenoids of hops to linalool, terpineol, and geraniol, which can stamp floral and fresh aromas to beers [110], has been reported.

Pichia kluyveri is another yeast species that may increase the levels of fruity acetate esters in beer [102]. In sequential fermentations with *S. cerevisiae*, a considerable enhancement was observed in the isoamyl acetate (banana-like flavor) concentration in a wheat beer production [111]. Another yeast species, *Wickerhamomyces anomalus*, whose characteristics have been further studied for winemaking, seems to have potential to be used for beer fermentations. Several strains were shown to present a wide range of enzymatic activities, including β-glucosidase activity, and they were shown to be good producers of esters, mainly ethyl acetate, and other fruity acetate esters, such as isoamyl acetate, contributing to improve aromatic complexity of fermented wort, likewise in co- or sequential inoculations with *S. cerevisiae* [112].

Regarding the efficiency in producing lactic acid and ethanol during wort fermentation, and the sensory characteristics, some isolates of the species *Hanseniaspora vineae, Lachancea fermentati, Lachancea thermotolerans, Schizosaccharomyces japonicus*, and *Wickerhamomyces anomalus* have been pointed out to be used for the production of sour beers in a single fermentation step, without the need of lactic acid bacteria for souring [113, 114]. This process was called primary souring, and the resulting beers showed both lactic tartness and fruity aromatic and flavor notes [114].

Several strains of nonconventional yeast species have been demonstrated to be useful in producing beers with reduced ethanol levels, besides contributing on improved sensory profile. The inability to consume the main brewery wort fermentable sugars, maltose and maltotriose, makes them less efficient at producing ethanol, enabling the production of low-alcohol (0.5–1.2% v/v) and alcohol-free (<0.5% v/v) beers [89, 115]. Pure cultures of several strains of *T. delbrueckii* were shown to ferment beers with an ethanol content varying from 0.9 to 2.6% (v/v) and characterized by rich fruity flavors [106, 108]. In the same way, strains of the species *Saccharomycodes ludwigii* stand out as suitable candidates, producing beers containing low alcohol concentration and higher amount of esters, besides lower diacetyl levels, contributing to mask the wort-like flavor, which is commonly identified in these kind of beers [115, 116]. Moreover, this yeast is already being used commercially to produce alcohol-free beers with increased fruity notes [115]. On the other hand, in a study aiming at screening basidiomycetous yeasts of *Mrakia* spp. for low alcohol beers, one strain of *M. gelida,* a psychrophilic one, was revealed to produce a more aromatic beer, judged to be fruitier with apricot, grape, and litchi descriptors, when compared with that produced by a commercial starter of *S. ludwigii* [117].

Other yeast strains of the species *Pichia kluyveri,* able to consume only glucose of brewing wort, were also shown to produce low-alcohol and alcohol-free beers with enhanced amounts of ester compounds and with a flavor profile similar to commercial standard beers of around 4% alcohol (v/v) [118]. One strain of *Williopsis saturnus* var. *mrakii* was demonstrated to have application in fermenting extra-fruity low-alcohol beers, due to the ability to increase the levels of acetate esters and to retain the terpenes and terpenoids of hopped wort, positively stamping fruity and floral flavors, besides preserving the hop aromas [119]. *Candida shehatae, C. tropicalis*, and *Zygosaccharomyces rouxii* are other species that have already been considered for the purpose of producing beers with low or no alcohol [89, 115].

The use of nonconventional yeasts in the brewing processes, especially considering the growth in the craft beer sector, stands out as natural and innovative choices to improve and bring differentiation to the beers. The potential of different yeast species to enrich and diversify the flavors and aromas, bringing sensory complexity to the beverages, recently comes out and should be more explored and studied as these abilities can result in peculiar beers, with unique features.

2.3 Coffee and cocoa fermentation

For satisfactory conduction of industrial fermentative processes, yeasts are applied in order to (I) reduce fermentation time, (II) generate end-products with high productivity, and (III) standardize processes. Concerning coffee and cocoa, yeast fermentation has not been well established. Recent studies pointed out that yeast fermentation can control cocoa and coffee fermentations and produce beans with improved quality. However, to reach a uniform level of high quality, similar to those obtained by fermentation processes of wines, beers, dairy products, and meat, the prerequisite is to know the different yeast groups that actively participate in these fermentation processes to draw a correlation of the final quality. The focus of this section is to describe the main nonconventional yeasts associated with the fermentation of coffee and cocoa beans and their role for each process.

During fermentation, depulped coffee beans are exposed to a diversity of microorganisms, such as yeasts, filamentous fungi, and bacteria that find favorable conditions for their development. The microbial activity generates a range of metabolites that can influence the final quality of the beverage [120, 121]. Yeasts are considered to be important due to pectin degradation and formation of flavor metabolites such as ethanol, organic acids, and esters. Due to these characteristics, many yeasts have been used as starter cultures for cocoa and coffee [122–124]. Different studies have demonstrated a high diversity of nonconventional yeasts during the coffee processing stage, including *Pichia kluyveri, P. anomala, P. guilliermondii, Kloeckera apiculata, Hanseniaspora uvarum, S. marxianus (Kluyveromyces marxianus), S. bayanus, Debaryomyces hansenii, D. polymorphus, Torulaspora delbrueckii, Torulopsis famata, Candida guilliermondii, C. parapsilosis, C. pelliculosa, C. famata, C. tropicalis, C. fermentati, C. membranifaciens, Rhodotorula mucilaginosa, Arxula adeninivorans, Cryptococcus albidus*, *Schizosaccharomyces* sp. and *Kloeckera* sp. [120–122, 125–128].

During coffee processing, the use of pectinolytic microorganisms is made to remove the mucilage layer from the coffee beans. This activity can significantly reduce fermentation time from 80 to 20 hours by enzymatic treatment. Thus, the production of pectinases has been the main attribution of yeasts and bacteria during coffee processing. Nonconventional yeasts, such as *P. anomala, P. kluyveri, P. Caribbean, P. guilliermondii*, and *H. uvarum,* have been associated with the production of pectinases during coffee fermentation [126]. The ability of yeasts belonging to the species *P. anomala, P. kluyveri*, and *H. uvarum* to produce pectic enzymes suggests that these species may act in the degradation of pectin during fruit fermentation [129].

Yeasts as starter cultures for the fermentation industry have been widespread by the ability to generate uniform and safe products, as well as the ability to modify various constituents related to organoleptic properties and nutritional, chemical, and microbiological characteristics. Most research on starter cultures for coffee fermentation has focused on selection of pectinolytic yeasts. Nonconventional yeasts, such as *P. guilliermondii* and *C. parapsilosis*, have revealed important pectinolytic potential [130]. In addition, yeasts such as *C. parapsilosis* and *S. cerevisiae* are coffee starters due to differentiated aroma production [131].

Researches with nonconventional yeasts in coffee fermentation have revealed the production of different volatile organic compounds. Different yeast species isolated from the dry and semi-dry processes of coffee produce significant amounts of aroma compounds (*e.g.*, acetoin, furfural, butyric acid, 2-phenyl-ethanone, 1,2-propanediol, hexanoic acid, decanoic acid, and nonanoic acid, among others), suggesting the strains *P. guilliermondii* UFLACN731 and *C. parapsilosis* UFLACN448 as promising candidates for coffee fermentation [130].

The importance of fermentation in the contribution of chocolate quality has been recognized for more than 90 years. Several studies and research have been conducted in different countries to determine the species of microorganisms associated with this process. A succession between yeast, lactic acid bacteria, and acetic acid bacteria is generally observed. This succession begins when high concentrations of sugars, low pH, and oxygen tension favor the growth of yeasts that convert the carbohydrates of the pulp into ethanol, dominating the process for approximately 48 hours. Lactic acid bacteria also ferment the sugars and utilize citric acid from the pulp; its growth is favored by the scarcity of oxygen and slight elevations of pH and temperature. With disintegration of the mucilaginous pulp surrounding the cocoa beans and together with the pH and aeration of mass, the citric acid present in the pulp is reduced by action of the yeasts, which favors the growth of acetic bacteria. These bacteria promote the oxidation of ethanol, initially produced by the yeast, to acetic acid in an extremely exothermic reaction, raising the temperature of the fermentative mass to levels of 45–50°C. The high temperature is important to enzymatic reactions, necessary for the development of the aroma and flavor of chocolate. Acetic acid, when penetrating cotyledonous tissues, promotes the death of the bean embryo (48–72 hours), and, together with ethanol, they act synergistically causing the diffusion of polyphenols in cotyledonary tissues. These reactions are important in the generation of well-fermented cocoa beans. Other microbial groups, such as *Bacillus* and filamentous fungi, develop in the final stages of fermentation, but the role of these microorganisms has not yet been fully elucidated [132–135].

To date, cocoa and coffee fermentations have been carried out with wild microorganisms present in the raw material and equipment used. Some studies have been carried out for the selection of cocoa and coffee cultures, where the main objective is to develop a faster fermentation process through the use of microorganisms producing pectinolytic enzymes. A study carried out cocoa fermentation inoculated with *Saccharomyces chevalieri* (now classified as *Saccharomyces cerevisiae*), *Candida zeylanoides*, and *Kluyveromyces fragilis* (now classified as *Kluyveromyces marxianus*) [136]. These yeasts were selected as being part of the natural flora of the cocoa fermentation environment and for producing pectinolytic enzymes. The fermentations inoculated with these yeasts were faster and produced chocolates with similar sensory characteristics in relation to spontaneously conducted fermentations [136].

The use of aromatic nonconventional yeasts, *P. kluyveri* and *K. marxianus,* during the cocoa fermentation process is able to alter the flavor profile of the chocolates compared to a spontaneously fermented control. The chocolates obtained after being submitted to this fermentation process can obtain higher grades in relation to the fruity flavor, cocoa aroma, and general taste. Some patents have been developed with the objective of establishing methods to optimize the cocoa fermentation process [137]. A method consisted of the addition of aromatic substances during the cocoa fermentation process with the aim of obtaining modified cocoa almonds. These substances comprise fruit pulp, aromatic leaves, and wood parts, among others [138]. *Pichia kluyveri* strain is a starter culture during cocoa fermentation adjusting the contents of isobutyl acetate and isoamyl acetate in obtained cocoa nibs. In addition, *P. kluyveri* demonstrated the ability to liquefy the cocoa pulp completely, due to its high pectinolytic activity [139].

2.4 Plant growth promotion

Throughout this chapter, the biotechnological potential of yeasts from other genera than *Saccharomyces* for activities and products commonly performed and generated by *Saccharomyces* spp. was discussed and exhibited. These activities are mainly associated with the industrial utilization of yeasts for the production of food, bioethanol, and alcoholic beverages through the fermentative metabolism. Nonconventional yeasts were initially shown to be able to generate high levels of a compound conventionally produced by *S. cerevisiae* (ethanol), but fermenting an alternative sugar (xylose) whose *Saccharomyces* spp. are naturally unable attracts interest in the bioenergy industry. Many of these strains are also able to generate a compound of industrial interest that *Saccharomyces* spp. cannot produce, *i.e.*, xylitol. Then, several strains of nonconventional yeasts able to replace *Saccharomyces* spp. in the industry of beer, coffee and chocolate were presented, which can improve aroma and flavors of these products. Yeasts are being unintentionally used by mankind for such purposes since the primitive beginning of microbial biotechnology. Therefore, food and bioenergy are the traditional fields of application of these unicellular fungi. However, the application of nonconventional yeasts is beyond the fields where *Saccharomyces* spp. are traditionally used. In this section, the potential application of nonconventional yeasts in a nonconventional field: agricultural biotechnology will be shown.

Many strains of nonconventional yeast species have been demonstrated as plant growth-promoting (PGP) microorganisms. PGP microorganisms live in the soil surrounding plant roots (rhizosphere), inside plant roots, stems and leaves (endophytes), or externally attached to plant surfaces (epiphytes) [140, 141]. The set of microbes inhabiting these many plant compartments is organized in microbial communities comprising the plant microbiome [140, 141]. The rhizosphere harbors a microbiome with higher diversity, abundance, and activity than the other plant compartments and is enriched in PGP microbes [142]. PGP microbes perform many activities that support plant growth and health, helping plants against biotic and abiotic stressors, besides directly acting in plant nutrition and growth regulation [142].

Inoculation of PGP microbes has the potential to replace the agrochemicals normally used in cropping systems, which can be expensive and environmentally harmful, and from nonrenewable sources [143]. The studies and applications of plant growth-promoting yeasts have lagged behind those of bacteria and other fungi [144, 145]. However, some studies showing beneficial activities of yeasts for plant productivity indicate that they can be as important as other microbes in agricultural biotechnology [146–148]. Some PGP features, as well as the main nonconventional yeast species able to perform these activities are discussed below.

Among the PGP activities performed by yeasts, biosynthesis of indole-3-acetic acid (IAA) is the most reported in the literature, found in many distinct yeast species and genera [144, 145, 147, 149–155]. IAA is a plant hormone of the auxin class, associated with phytostimulation by increasing root growth [156, 157]. In the *Rhodotorula* genus, two species were identified as able to produce IAA in many studies. *R. graminis* is a yeast species isolated from the internal tissues of poplar tree and able to produce high amounts of IAA [149]. This capacity results in the growth promotion of distinct plants, such as poplar itself, as well as pepper and maize [150–152]. A genome survey did not detect the genes involved in the conventional pathways of IAA biosynthesis and suggested putative genes for alternative pathways in this species [154]. Strains of the species *R. mucilaginosa*, isolated from poplar stems or from soils cropped with legumes, were also found as high IAA producers [149, 155]. Experiments using this species indicated its growth promotion activity in poplar and tomato [150–152].

Candida tropicalis is another important yeast species isolated from the rhizosphere of rice and maize, whose ability to synthesize IAA besides other PGP activities was shown to promote growth of these mentioned crops [145, 153]. Other examples of IAA biosynthesizing yeast species are *Aureobasidium pullulans*, *Cryptococcus flavus*, *Hannaella sinensis*, *Rhodosporidium paludigenum*, *Torulaspora globosa*, and *Williopsis saturnus* [144, 147, 155].

Another important PGP activity performed by some yeast species is phosphate solubilization and interaction with mycorrhizal fungi able to mobilize phosphate to plants [153, 158, 159]. Phosphorus (P) is a macroelement required by plants in high levels. Plants cropped in soils with low availability of phosphate are highly benefited from the activity of P-solubilizing microbes for their nutrition. These PGP microbes produce organic acids that release the phosphate attached to mineral surfaces, making this nutrient available for root absorption [160].

The yeast species *Yarrowia lipolytica*, *Torulaspora globosa*, and *Candida tropicalis* were shown as able to solubilize inorganic phosphate in *in vitro* tests [147, 153, 160]. Some strains of the species *Candida railenensis* and *Cryptococcus flavus* were not able to directly solubilize phosphate, but exhibited a microbial interaction with arbuscular mycorrhizal fungi resulting in higher P-solubilization and promotion of maize growth [159]. On the other hand, another study observed that yeast strains from the genera *Rhodotorula* and *Cryptococcus* were able to both interact with the mycorrhizal fungus *Glomus mosseae* and solubilize phosphate [158].

The agricultural productivity of many crops is highly impaired by plant diseases, mainly caused by fungal pathogens. Use of PGP microbes that perform biocontrol of these fungi is a promising alternative to the use of expensive and bioaccumulative fungicides [143]. The capacity of pathogen biocontrol is present in many nonconventional yeast species that perform different types of antagonism, including competition for space and nutrients, antibiosis, fungal cell wall degradation, mycoparasitism and induction of host resistance [146].

Strains of the species *Candida valida*, *Rhodotorula glutinis*, and *Trichosporon asahii*, isolated from the sugar beet rhizosphere, were shown to control the fungus *Rhizoctonia solani* that causes root damping-off, promoting growth and health of this plant [161]. Another strain of *R. glutinis* was isolated from the inner tissues of the apple fruit and was able to promote growth of apple tree by controlling the pathogen *Botrytis cinerea* [162]. The species of the genus *Rhodotorula* commonly produce a siderophore called rhodoturulic acid, which inhibits *B. cinerea* spore germination. Utilization of *R. glutinis* in combination with the application of rhodoturulic acid resulted in a more efficient control of *B. cinerea* [162]. Other yeast species like *Hannaella sinensis* and *Rhodosporidium paludigenum* produce different siderophores, but the analyzed strains of these species showed no antifungal activity [147].

An epiphyte yeast strain of the species *Torulaspora globosa* isolated from rice leaf surface is antagonistic to many fungi causing plant diseases, including *Fusarium moniliforme*, *Helminthosporium oryzae*, and *Rhizoctonia solani* [147]. In addition to efficient biocontrol, this strain synthesizes IAA, indicating its high potential to be used as an agricultural inoculant [147]. Strains of the species *Aureobasidium pullulans* and *Rhodotorula mucilaginosa*, isolated from soils cropped with legumes, showed antagonism to the fungi *Phytophthora infestans* and *Fusarium graminearum*, respectively [155].

In addition to the three mentioned PGP activities previously shown, *i.e.* IAA biosynthesis, P-solubilization and biocontrol, many others are present in nonconventional yeasts. For example, yeasts can help plants against several types of stress. The compound 1-aminocyclopropane-1-carboxylic acid (ACC) is a precursor in ethylene biosynthesis. High ethylene levels are induced in plants facing many types of stress [163]. PGP microbes that produce the enzyme ACC deaminase decrease the levels of ethylene, alleviating plant stress and indirectly promoting their growth [163]. Despite this activity is more present in bacteria, the yeast species *Candida tropicalis*, also capable of P-solubilization and IAA biosynthesis, was shown to produce ACC deaminase, which possibly contributed to rice growth promotion in pot experiments [145]. The biotechnological potential of the strain *C. tropicalis* HY was validated with the inclusion of this strain in the commercial biofertilizer product BioGro, which improves paddy rice yield [145].

Other type of common stress in plants is the oxidative. Reactive oxygen species such as hydrogen peroxide (H_2O_2) can damage plant tissues. The accumulation of these compounds can be mitigated by the activity of the enzyme catalase. Although this PGP function is also more observed in bacteria, some yeasts that use methanol as carbon and energy sources contains catalases, since H_2O_2 is a by-product of that metabolism [147]. Strains of *Cryptococcus flavus*, *Hannaella sinensis*, *Rhodosporidium paludigenum*, and *Torulaspora globosa* produce catalase and thus can potentially help plants against the oxidative stress, in addition to the PGP activities already described for these species [147].

The biotechnological utilization of PGP microbes in agriculture is in its infancy, since much knowledge and technology must be developed in order to efficiently replace agrochemicals. Nonconventional yeasts were shown to perform many beneficial activities to plants and need to be explored more to increase their utilization together with PGP bacteria and filamentous fungi for a more sustainable agriculture.

Conflict of interest

The authors declare that they have no competing interests.

Author details

Camila de Souza Varize[1*], Renata Maria Christofoleti-Furlan[1], Elisangela de Souza Miranda Muynarsk[2], Gilberto Vinícius de Melo Pereira[2], Lucas Dantas Lopes[1] and Luiz Carlos Basso[1]

1 Departament of Biological Sciences, "Luiz de Queiroz" College of Agriculture, University of São Paulo, Piracicaba, SP, Brazil

2 Department of Bioprocess Engineering and Biotechnology, Federal University of Parana, Curitiba, PR, Brazil

*Address all correspondence to: camilasv@usp.br

References

[1] Reed G. Yeast technology—Introduction. In: Reed G, Yeast Technology. 1st ed. The Netherlands: Springer; 1991. pp. 1-5. DOI: 10.1007/978-94-011-9771-7

[2] Legras JL, Merdinoglu D, Cornuet JM, Karst F. Bread, beer and wine: Saccharomyces cerevisiae diversity reflects human history. Molecular Ecology. 2007;**16**(10):2091-2102. DOI: 10.1111/j.1365-294X.2007.03266.x

[3] Wu J, Elliston A, Le-Gall G, Colquhoun IJ, Collins SRA, Dicks J, et al. Yeast diversity in relation to the production of fuels and chemicals. Scientific Reports. 2017;**7**(14259):1-11. DOI: 10.1038/s41598-017-14641-0

[4] Sicard D, Legras JL. Bread, beer and wine: Yeast domestication in the Saccharomyces sensu stricto complex. Comptes Rendus Biologies. 2011;**334**(3):229-236. DOI: 10.1016/j.crvi.2010.12.016

[5] Hittinger CT, Rokas A, Bai FY, Boekhout T, Gonçalves P, Jeffries TW, et al. Genomics and the making of yeast biodiversity. Current Opinion in Genetics & Development. 2015;**35**:100-109. DOI: 10.1016/j.gde.2015.10.008

[6] Dujon BA, Louis EJ. Genome diversity and evolution in the budding yeasts (Saccharomycotina). Genetics. 2017;**206**(2):717-750. DOI: 10.1534/genetics.116.199216

[7] Hittinger CT, Steele JL, Ryder DS. Diverse yeasts for diverse fermented beverages and foods. Current Opinion in Biotechnology. 2018;**49**:199-206. DOI: 10.1016/j.copbio.2017.10.004

[8] Weber H, Barth G. Nonconventional yeasts: Their genetics and biotechnological applications. Critical Reviews in Biotechnology. 1988;**7**(4):281-337. DOI: 10.3109/07388558809150535

[9] Spencer J, Spencer AR, Laluce C. Non-conventional yeasts. Applied Microbiology and Biotechnology. 2002;**58**(2):147-156. DOI: 10.1007/s00253-001-0834-2

[10] Domínguez A, Fermiñán E, Sánchez M, González FJ, Pérez-Campo FM, García S, et al. Non-conventional yeasts as hosts for heterologous protein production. International Microbiology. 1998;**1**(2):131-142

[11] Gao M, Cao M, Suástegui M, Walker J, Rodriguez-Quiroz N, Wu Y, et al. Innovating a nonconventional yeast platform for producing shikimate as the building block of high-value aromatics. ACS Synthetic Biology (ACS Publications). 2017;**6**(1):29-38. DOI: 10.1021/acssynbio.6b00132

[12] Bleve G, Lezzi C, Chiriatti MA, D'Ostuni I, Tristezza M, Di Venere D, et al. Selection of non-conventional yeasts and their use in immobilized form for the bioremediation of olive oil mill wastewaters. Bioresource Technology. 2011;**102**(2):982-989. DOI: 10.1016/j.biortech.2010.09.059

[13] Türker M. Yeast biotechnology: Diversity and applications. Advances in science and industrial productions of Baker's yeast. In: Conference: Proceedings of 27th VH Yeast Conference; 14-15 April 2014; Istanbul. 2014. pp. 1-26

[14] Walker GM. Yeast technology. In: Walker GM, editor. Yeast Physiology and Biotechnology. 1st ed. West Sussex: John Wiley & Sons Ltd; 1998. pp. 265-308. ISBN-10: 0471964468

[15] Nigan P, Singh D. Processes for fermentative production of xylitol—A sugar substitute. Process Biochemistry. 1995;**30**(2):117-124. DOI: 10.1016/0032-9592(95)80001-8

[16] Searchinger T, Heimlich R, Houghton RA, Dong F, Elobeid A,

Fabiosa J, et al. Use of U.S. croplands for biofuels increases greenhouse gases through emissions from land-use change. Science. 2008;**319**(5867):1238-1240. DOI: 10.1126/science.1151861

[17] Sathre R. Comparing the heat of combustion of fossil fuels to the heat accumulated by their lifecycle greenhouse gases. Fuel. 2014;**115**: 647-677. DOI: 10.1016/j.fuel.2013.07.069

[18] Hook M, Tang X. Depletion of fossil fuels and anthropogenic climate change—A review. Energy Policy. 2013;**52**:797-809. DOI: 10.1016/j.enpol.2012.10.046

[19] Ragauskas AJ, Williams CK, Davison BH, Britovsek G, Cairney J, Eckert CA, et al. The path forward for biofuels and biomaterials. Science. 2006;**311**(5760):484-489. DOI: 10.1126/science.1114736

[20] Sánchez OJ, Cardona CA. Trends in biotechnological production of fuel ethanol from different feedstocks. Bioresource Technology. 2008;**99**(13):5270-5295. DOI: 10.1016/j.biortech.2007.11.013

[21] Gerbens-Leenes PW, van-Lienden AR, Hoekstra AY, van der Meer TH. Biofuel scenarios in a water perspective: The global blue and green water footprint of road transport in 2030. Global Environmental Change. 2012;**22**(3):764-775. DOI: 10.1016/j.gloenvcha.2012.04.001

[22] Koçar G, Civas N. An overview of biofuels from energy crops: Current status and future prospects. Renewable and Sustainable Energy Reviews. 2013;**28**:900-916. DOI: 10.1016/j.rser.2013.08.022

[23] Sarkar N, Ghosh SK, Bannerjee S, Aikat K. Bioethanol production from agricultural wastes: An overview. Renewable Energy. 2012;**37**(1):19-27. DOI: 10.1016/j.renene.2011.06.045

[24] Wiselogel A, Tyson S, Johnson D. Biomass feedstock resources and composition. In: Wyman CE, editor. Handbook on Bioethanol: Production and Utilization. 1st ed. Washington: Taylor & Francis; 1996. pp. 105-118. ISBN: 1560325534, 9781560325536

[25] Rubin EM. Genomics of cellulosic biofuels. Nature. 2008;**454**(14):841-845. DOI: 10.1038/nature07190

[26] Saha BC. Lignocellulose biodegradation and applications in biotechnology. In: Saha BC, Hayashi K, editors. Lignocellulose Biodegradation. 1st ed. Washington: American Chemical Society; 2004. pp. 2-25. ISBN: 0841238766, 9780841238763

[27] O'neill MA, York WS. The composition and structure of plant primary cell walls. In: Rose JKC, editor. The Plant Cell Wall. 1st ed. Oxford: Blackwell Publishing; 2003. pp. 1-54. ISBN: 9781841273280

[28] Lachke A. Biofuel from D-xylose—The second most abundant sugar. Resonance. 2002;7(5):50-58. DOI: 10.1007/BF02836736

[29] Kuhad RC, Gupta R, Khasa YP, Singh A, Zhang YHP. Bioethanol production from pentose sugars: Current status and future prospects. Renewable and Sustainable Energy Reviews. 2011;**15**(9):4950-4962. DOI: 10.1016/j.rser.2011.07.058

[30] Chu BCH, Lee H. Genetic improvement of *Saccharomyces cerevisiae* for xylose fermentation. Biotechnology Advances. 2007;**25**(5):425-441. DOI: 10.1016/j.biotechadv.2007.04.001

[31] Batt CA, Caryallo S, Easson DD Jr, Akedo M, Sinskey AJ. Direct evidence for a xylose metabolic pathway in *Saccharomyces cerevisiae*. Biotechnology and Bioengineering. 1986;**28**(4): 549-553. DOI: 10.1002/bit.260280411

[32] Hahn-Hagerdal B, Karhumaa K, Fonseca C, Spencer-Martins I, Gorwa-Grauslund MF. Towards industrial pentose-fermenting yeast strains. Applied Microbiology and Biotechnology. 2007;**74**(5):937-953. DOI: 10.1007/s00253-006-0827-2

[33] Mãkinen KK. Can the pentitol-hexitol theory explain the clinical observations made with xylitol? Medical Hypotheses. 2000;**54**(4):603-613. DOI: 10.1054/mehy.1999.0904

[34] Nolleau V, Preziosi-Belloy JP, Delgenes JP, Navarro JM. Xylitol production from xylose by two yeast strains: Sugar tolerance. Current Microbiology. 1993;**27**(4):191-197. DOI: 10.1007/BF01692875

[35] Peterson ME. Xylitol. Topics in companion animal medicine. 2013;**28**(1):18-20. DOI: 10.1053/j.tcam.2013.03.008

[36] Dominguez JM, Gong CS, Tsao GT. Production of xylitol from D-xylose by *Debaryomyces hanseni*. Applied Biochemistry and Biotechnology. 1997;**63-65**:117-127. DOI: 10.1007/BF02920418

[37] Winkelhausen E, Kuzmanova S. Microbial conversion of D-xylose to xylitol. Journal of Fermentation and Bioengineering. 1998;**86**(1):1-14. DOI: 10.1016/S0922-338X(98)80026-3

[38] Misra S, Gupta P, Raghuwanshi S, Dutt K, Saxena RK. Comparative study on different strategies involved for xylitol purification from culture media fermented by *Candida tropicalis*. Separation and Purification Technology. 2011;**78**(3):266-273. DOI: 10.1016/j.seppur.2011.02.018

[39] Mussato SI, Roberto IC. Xilitol: Edulcorante com efeitos benéficos para a saúde humana. Revista Brasileira de Ciências Farmacêuticas. 2002;**38**(4):401-413. DOI: 10.1590/S1516-93322002000400003

[40] Guo C, Zhao C, He P, Lu D, Shen A, Jiang N. Screening and characterization of yeasts for xylitol production. Journal of Applied Microbiology. 2006;**101**:1096-1104. DOI: 10.1111/j.1365-2672.2006.02994.x

[41] West TP. Xylitol production by *Candida* species grown on a grass hydrolysate. World Journal of Microbiology and Biotechnology. 2009;**25**:913-916. DOI: 10.1007/s11274-008-9947-4

[42] Jeffries TW, Kurtzman CP. Strain selection, taxonomy, and genetics of xylose-fermenting yeasts. Enzyme and Microbial Technology. 1994;**16**:922-932. DOI: 10.1016/0141-0229(94)90001-9

[43] Schneider H, Wang PY, Chan YK, Maleszka R. Conversion of D-xylose into ethanol by the yeast *Pachysolen tannophilus*. Biotechnology Letters. 1981;**3**(2):89-92. DOI: 10.1002/bit.260240210

[44] Morikawa Y, Takasawa S, Masunaga I, Takayama K. Ethanol productions from D-xylose and cellobiose by *Kluyveromyces cellobiovorus*. Biotechnology and Bioengineering. 1985;**27**(4):509-513. DOI: 10.1002/bit.260270417

[45] Du Preez JC, Bosch M, Prior BA. Xylose fermentation by *Candida shehatae* and *Picchia stipitis*: Effects of pH, temperature and substrate concentration. Enzyme and Microbial Technology. 1986;**8**(6):360-364. DOI: 10.1016/0141-0229(86)90136-5

[46] Agbogbo FK, Haagensen FD, Milam D, Wenger KS. Fermentation of acid-pretreated corn stover to ethanol without detoxification using *Pichia stipitis*. Applied Biochemistry and Biotechnology. 2008;**145**(1):53-58. DOI: 10.1007/s12010-007-8056-4

[47] Krahulec S, Kratzer R, Longus K, Nidetzky B. Comparison of

Scheffersomyces stipitis strains CBS5773 and CBS6054 with regard to their xylose metabolism: Implications for xylose fermentation. Microbiology Open. 2012;**1**(1):64-70. DOI: 10.1002/mbo3.5

[48] Cadete RM, Santos RO, Melo MA, Mouro A, Gonçalves DL, Stambuk BU, et al. *Spathaspora arborariae* sp. nov., a D-xylose-fermenting yeast species isolated from rotting wood in Brazil. FEMS Yeast Research. 2009;**9**(8):1338-1342. DOI: 10.1111/j.1567-1364.2009.00582.x

[49] Cunha-Pereira F, Hickert LR, Sehnem NT, de Souza-Cruz PB, Rosa CA, Ayub MA. Conversion of sugars present in rice hull hydrolysates into ethanol by *Spathaspora arborariae*, *Saccharomyces cerevisiae*, and their co-fermentations. Bioresource Technology. 2011;**102**(5):4218-4225. DOI: 10.1016/j.biortech.2010.12.060

[50] Cadete RM, de Las-Heras AM, Sandström AG, Ferreira C, Gírio F, Gorwa-Grauslund MF, et al. Exploring xylose metabolism in *Spathaspora* species: XYL1.2 from *Spathaspora passalidarum* as the key for efficient anaerobic xylose fermentation in metabolic engineered *Saccharomyces cerevisiae*. Biotechnology for Biofuels. 2016;**9**(167):1-14. DOI: 10.1186/s13068-016-0570-6

[51] Nguyen NH, Suh SO, Marshall CJ, Blackwell M. Morphological and ecological similarities: Wood-boring beetles associated with novel xylose-fermenting yeasts, *Spathaspora passalidarum* gen. sp. nov. and *Candida jeffriesii* sp. nov. Mycological Research. 2006;**110**(10):1232-1241. DOI: 10.1016/j.mycres.2006.07.002

[52] Hou X. Anaerobic xylose fermentation by *Spathaspora passalidarum*. Applied Microbiology and Biotechnology. 2012;**94**(1):205-214. DOI: 10.1007/s00253-011-3694-4

[53] Cadete RM, Melo MA, Dussán KJ, Rodrigues RCLB, Silva SS, Zilli JE, et al. Diversity and physiological characterization of D-xylose-fermenting yeasts isolated from the brazilian amazonian forest. PLoS One. 2012;**7**(8):1-11. DOI: 10.1371/journal.pone.0043135

[54] Varize CS, Cadete RM, Lopes LD, Christofoleti-Furlan RM, Lachance MA, Rosa CA, et al. *Spathaspora piracicabensis* f. a., sp. nov., a D-xylose-fermenting yeast species isolated from rotting wood in Brazil. Antonie Van Leeuwenhoek. 2018;**111**(4):525-531. DOI: 10.1007/s10482-017-0974-8

[55] Cadete RM, Rosa CA. The yeasts of the genus *Spathaspora*: Potential candidates for second-generation biofuel production. Yeast. 2018;**35**(2):191-199. DOI: 10.1002/yea.3279

[56] Jeffries TW. Conversion of xylose to ethanol under aerobic conditions by *Candida tropicalis*. Biotechnology Letters, Dordrecht. 1981;**3**(5):213-218. DOI: 10.1007/BF00154647

[57] Skoog K, Hahn-Hagerdal B. Xylose fermentation. Enzyme and Microbial Technology. 1988;**10**(2):66-80. DOI: 10.1016/0141-0229(88)90001-4

[58] Olsson L, Hahn-Hagerdal B. Fermentation of lignocellulosic hydrolysates for ethanol production. Enzyme and Microbial Technology. 1996;**18**:312-331. DOI: 10.1016/0141-0229(95)00157-3

[59] Chandra RP, Bura R, Mabee WE, Berlin A, Pan X, Saddler JN. Substrate pretreatment: The key to effective enzymatic hydrolysis of lignocellulosics? Advances in Biochemical Engineering/Biotechnology. 2007;**108**:67-93. DOI: 10.1007/10_2007_064

[60] Nogué VS, Karhumaa K. Xylose fermentation as a challenge for commercialization of lignocellulosic

fuels and chemicals. Biotechnology Letters. 2015;**37**(4):761-772. DOI: 10.1007/s10529-014-1756-2

[61] Hahn-Hagerdal B, Jeppsson H, Skoog K, Prior BA. Biochemistry and physiology of xylose fermentation by yeasts. Enzyme and Microbial Technology. 1994;**16**:933-943. DOI: 10.1016/0141-0229(94)90002-7

[62] Webb SR, Lee H. Regulation of D-xylose utilization by hexoses in pentose-fermenting yeasts. Biotechnology Advances. 1990;**8**(4):685-697. DOI: 10.1016/0734-9750(90)91991-O

[63] Pace NR. A molecular view of microbial diversity and the biosphere. Science. 1997;**276**(5313):734-740. DOI: 10.1126/science.276.5313.734

[64] Quince C, Curtis TP, Sloan WT. The rational exploration of microbial diversity. The ISME Journal—Nature. 2008;**2**(10):997-1006. DOI: 10.1038/ismej.2008.69

[65] Urbina H, Schuster J, Blackwell M. The gut of Guatemalan passalid beetles: A habitat colonized by cellobiose- and xylose-fermenting yeasts. Fungal Ecology. 2013;**6**(5):339-355. DOI: 10.1016/j.funeco.2013.06.005

[66] Wang Y, Ren YC, Zhang ZT, Ke T, Hui FL. *Spathaspora allomyrinae* sp. nov., a D-xylose-fermenting yeast species isolated from a scarabeid beetle *Allomyrina dichotoma*. International Journal of Systematic and Evolutionary Microbiology. 2016;**66**(5):2008-2012. DOI: 10.1099/ijsem.0.000979

[67] Martiniano SE, Chandel AK, Soares LC, Pagnocca FC, da Silva SS. Evaluation of novel xylose-fermenting yeast strains from Brazilian forests for hemicellulosic ethanol production from sugarcane bagasse. 3 Biotech. 2013;**3**(5):345-352. DOI: 10.1007/s13205-013-0145-1

[68] Martiniano SE, Philippini RR, Chandel AK, Rosa CA, Pagnocca FC, da Silva SS. Evaluation of rice bran extract as a nitrogen source for improved hemicellulosic ethanol production from sugarcane bagasse by new xylose-fermenting yeast strains isolated from Brazilian forests. Sugar Tech. 2014;**16**(1):1-8. DOI: 10.1007/s12355-013-0219-8

[69] Barretto DA, Avchar R, Carvalho C, Sampaio JP, Vootla SK, Baghela A. *Blastobotrys bombycis* sp. nov., a D-xylose-fermenting yeast isolated from the gut of the silkworm larva *Bombyx mori*. International Journal of Systematic and Evolutionary Microbiology. 2018;**68**(8):2638-2643. DOI: 10.1099/ijsem.0.002890

[70] Nitiyon S, Khunnamwong P, Lertwattanasakul N, Limtong S. *Candida kantuleensis* sp. nov., a D-xylose-fermenting yeast species isolated from peat in a tropical peat Swamp Forest. International Journal of Systematic and Evolutionary Microbiology. 2018;**68**(7):2313-2318. DOI: 10.1099/ijsem.0.002835

[71] Cadete RM, Fonseca C, Rosa CA. Novel yeast strains from Brazilian biodiversity: Biotechnological applications in lignocellulose conversion into biofuels. In: Silva SS, Chandel AK, editors. Biofuels in Brazil: Fundamental Aspects, Recent Developments, and Future Perspectives. 1st ed. Switzerland: Springer International Publishing; 2014. pp. 225-279. DOI: 10.1007/978-3-319-05020-1_12

[72] Jeffries TW, Grigoriev IV, Grimwood J, Laplaza JM, Aerts A, Salamov A, et al. Genome sequence of the lignocellulose-bioconverting and xylose-fermenting yeast *Pichia stipitis*. Nature Biotechnology. 2007;**25**(3): 319-326. DOI: 10.1038/nbt1290

[73] Lobo FP, Gonçalves DL, Alves SL Jr, Gerber AL, de Vasconcelos AT, Basso

LC, et al. Draft genome sequence of the D-xylose-fermenting yeast *Spathaspora arborariae* UFMG-HM19.1AT. Genome Announcements. 2014;**2**(1):1-2. DOI: 10.1128/genomeA.01163-13

[74] Lopes DD, Cibulski SP, Mayer FQ, Siqueira FM, Rosa CA, Hector RE, et al. Draft genome sequence of the D-xylose-fermenting yeast *Spathaspora xylofermentans* UFMG-HMD23.3. Genome Announcements. 2017;**5**(33): 1-2. DOI: 10.1128/genomeA.00815-17

[75] Spencer-Martins I. Transport of sugars in yeasts: Implications in the fermentation of lignocellulosic materials. Bioresource Technology. 1994;**50**(1):51-57. DOI: 10.1016/0960-8524(94)90220-8

[76] Lonn A, Traff-Bjerre KL, Otero RRC, van Zyl WH, Hahn-Hagerdal B. Xylose isomerase activity influences xylose fermentation with recombinant *Saccharomyces cerevisiae* strains expressing mutated *xylA* from *Thermus thermophilus*. Enzyme and Microbial Technology. 2003;**32**(5):567-573. DOI: 10.1016/S0141-0229(03)00024-3

[77] Jeffries TW. Engineering yeasts for xylose metabolism. Current Opinion in Biotechnology. 2005;**17**(3):320-326. DOI: 10.1016/j.copbio.2006.05.008

[78] van Dijken JP, Scheffers WA. Redox balances in the metabolism of sugars by yeasts. FEMS Microbiology Letters. 1986;**32**(3-4):199-224. DOI: 10.1016/0378-1097(86)90291-0

[79] Du Preez JC. Process parameters and environmental factors affecting D-xylose fermentation by yeasts. Enzyme and Microbial Technology. 1994;**16**(11):944-956. DOI: 10.1016/0141-0229(94)90003-5

[80] Furlan SA, Bouilloud P, Castro HF. Influence of oxygen on ethanol and xylitol production by xylose fermenting yeasts. Process Biochemistry. 1994;**29**(8):657-662. DOI: 10.1016/0032-9592(94)80043-X

[81] Ikeuchi T, Azuma M, Kato J, Ooshima H. Screening of microorganisms for xylitol production and fermentation behavior in high concentrations of xylose. Biomass and Bioenergy. 1999;**16**(5):333-339. DOI: 10.1016/S0961-9534(99)00005-7

[82] Tamburini E, Bianchini E, Bruni A, Forlani G. Cosubstrate effect on xylose reductase and xylitol dehydrogenase activity levels, and its consequence on xylitol production by *Candida tropicalis*. Enzyme and Microbial Technology. 2010;**46**(5):352-359. DOI: 10.1016/j.enzmictec.2010.01.001

[83] Bruinenberg PM. The NADP(H) redox couple in yeast metabolism. Antonie Van Leeuwenhoek. 1986;**52**(5):411-429. DOI: 10.1007/BF00393469

[84] Rizzi M, Harwart K, Bui-Thanh NA, Dellweg H. A kinetic study of the NAD^+-xylitol-dehydrogenase from the yeast *Pichia stipitis*. Journal of Fermentation and Bioengineering. 1989;**67**(1):25-30. DOI: 10.1016/0922-338X(89)90081-0

[85] Zeng QK, Du HL, Wang JF, Wei DQ, Wang XN. Reversal of coenzyme specificity and improvement of catalytic efficiency of *Pichia stipitis* xylose reductase by rational site-directed mutagenesis. Biotechnology Letters. 2009;**31**(7):1025-1029. DOI: 10.1007/s10529-009-9980-x

[86] Pal S, Choudhary V, Kumar A, Biswas D, Mondal AK, Sahoo DK. Studies on xylitol production by metabolic pathway engineered *Debaryomyces hansenii*. Bioresource Technology. 2013;**147**:449-455. DOI: 10.1016/j.biortech.2013.08.065

[87] Madhavan A, Tamalampudi S, Ushida K, Kanai D, Katahira S, Srivastava A, et al. Xylose isomerase

from polycentric fungus *Orpinomyces*: Gene sequencing, cloning, and expression in *Saccharomyces cerevisiae* for bioconversion of xylose to ethanol. Applied Microbiology and Biotechnology. 2009;**82**(6):1067-1078. DOI: 10.1007/s00253-008-1794-6

[88] Steensels J, Verstrepen KJ. Taming wild yeast: Potential of conventional and nonconventional yeasts in industrial fermentations. Annual Review of Microbiology. 2014;**68**(1):61-80. DOI: 10.1146/annurev-micro-091213-113025

[89] Michel M, Meier-Dörnberg T, Jacob F, Methner FJ, Wagner RS, Hutzler M. Review: Pure non-*Saccharomyces* starter cultures for beer fermentation with a focus on secondary metabolites and practical applications. Journal of the Institute of Brewing. 2016;**122**:569-587. DOI: 10.1002/jib.381

[90] Gibson B, Geertman JMA, Hittinger CT, Krogerus K, Libkind D, Louis EJ, et al. New yeasts-new brews: Modern approaches to brewing yeast design and development. FEMS Yeast Research. 2017;**17**(4):1-13. DOI: 10.1093/femsyr/fox038

[91] Jolly NP, Varela C, Pretorius IS. Not your ordinary yeast: Non-*Saccharomyces* yeasts in wine production uncovered. FEMS Yeast Research. 2014;**14**(2):215-237. DOI: 10.1111/1567-1364.12111

[92] Bokulich NA, Bamforth CW. The microbiology of malting and brewing. Microbiology and Molecular Biology Reviews. 2013;**77**:157-172. DOI: 10.1128/MMBR.00060-12

[93] Capece A, Romaniello R, Siesto G, Romano P. Conventional and non-conventional yeasts in beer production. Fermentation. 2018;**4**:38. DOI: 10.3390/fermentation4020038

[94] Vanderhaegen B, Neven H, Coghe S, Verstrepen KJ, Derdelinckx G, Verachtert H. Bioflavoring and beer refermentation. Applied Microbiology and Biotechnology. 2003;**62**(2-3):140-150. DOI: 10.1007/s00253-003-1340-5

[95] Basso RF, Alcarde AR, Portugal CB. Could non-*Saccharomyces* yeasts contribute on innovative brewing fermentations? Food Research International. 2016;**86**:112-120. DOI: 10.1016/j.foodres.2016.06.002

[96] Bokulich NA, Bamforth CW, Mills DA. Brewhouse-resident microbiota are responsible for multi-stage fermentation of American coolship ale. PLoS One. 2012;**7**(4):e35507. DOI: 10.1371/journal.pone.0035507

[97] Spitaels F, Wieme AD, Janssens M, Aerts M, Daniel HM, Van Landschoot A, et al. The microbial diversity of traditional spontaneously fermented lambic beer. PLoS One. 2014;**9**(4):e95384. DOI: 10.1371/journal.pone.0095384

[98] Varela C. The impact of non-*Saccharomyces* yeasts in the production of alcoholic beverages. Applied Microbiology and Biotechnology. 2016;**100**(23):9861-9874. DOI: 10.1007/s00253-016-7941-6

[99] Colomer MS, Funch B, Forster J. The raise of *Brettanomyces* yeast species for beer production. Current Opinion in Biotechnology. 2018;**56**:30-35. DOI: 10.1016/j.copbio.2018.07.009

[100] Steensels J, Daenen L, Malcorps P, Derdelinckx G, Verachtert H, Verstrepen KJ. *Brettanomyces* yeasts—From spoilage organisms to valuable contributors to industrial fermentations. International Journal of Food Microbiology. 2015;**206**:24-38. DOI: 10.1016/j.ijfoodmicro.2015.04.005

[101] Godoy L, Martínez C, Carrasco N, Ganga MA. Purification and characterization of a p-coumarate decarboxylase and a vinylphenol

reductase from *Brettanomyces bruxellensis*. International Journal of Food Microbiology. 2008;**127**:6-11. DOI: 10.1016/j.ijfoodmicro.2008.05.011

[102] Holt S, Mukherjee V, Lievens B, Verstrepen KJ, Thevelein JM. Bioflavoring by non-conventional yeasts in sequential beer fermentations. Food Microbiology. 2018;**72**:55-66. DOI: 10.1016/J.FM.2017.11.008

[103] Lentz M, Harris C. Analysis of growth inhibition and metabolism of hydroxycinnamic acids by brewing and spoilage strains of *Brettanomyces* yeast. Food. 2015;**4**:581-593. DOI: 10.3390/foods4040581

[104] Kuo HP, Wang R, Huang CY, Lai JT, Lo YC, Huang ST. Characterization of an extracellular β-glucosidase from *Dekkera bruxellensis* for resveratrol production. Journal of Food and Drug Analysis. 2018;**26**:163-171. DOI: 10.1016/j.jfda.2016.12.016

[105] Toh DWK, Chua JY, Liu SQ. Impact of simultaneous fermentation with *Saccharomyces cerevisiae* and *Torulaspora delbrueckii* on volatile and non-volatile constituents in beer. Food Science and Technology. 2018;**91**:26-33. DOI: 10.1016/j.lwt.2018.01.025

[106] Canonico L, Agarbati A, Comitini F, Ciani M. *Torulaspora delbrueckii* in the brewing process: A new approach to enhance bioflavour and to reduce ethanol content. Food Microbiology. 2016;**56**:45-51. DOI: 10.1016/j.fm.2015.12.005

[107] Canonico L, Comitini F, Ciani M. *Torulaspora delbrueckii* contribution in mixed brewing fermentations with different *Saccharomyces cerevisiae* strains. International Journal of Food Microbiology. 2017;**259**:7-13. DOI: 10.1016/j.ijfoodmicro.2017.07.017

[108] Michel M, Kopecká J, Meier-Dörnberg T, Zarnkow M, Jacob F, Hutzler M. Screening for new brewing yeasts in the non-*Saccharomyces* sector with *Torulaspora delbrueckii* as model. Yeast. 2016;**33**:129-144. DOI: 10.1002/yea.3146

[109] Tataridis P, Kanellis A, Logothetis S, Nerantzis E. Use of non-*Saccharomyces Torulaspora delbrueckii* yeast strains in winemaking and brewing. Journal of Natural Science. 2013;**124**:415-426. DOI: 10.2298/ZMSPN1324415T

[110] King A, Dickinson JR. Biotransformation of monoterpene alcohols by *Saccharomyces cerevisiae*, *Torulaspora delbrueckii* and *Kluyveromyces lactis*. Yeast. 2000;**16**(6):499-506. DOI: 10.1002/(SICI)1097-0061(200004)16:6<499::AID-YEA548>3.0.CO;2-E

[111] Saerens S, Swiegers JH. Enhancement of beer flavor by a combination of *Pichia* yeast and different hop varieties. 2013. Patent number: WO2013/030398A1

[112] Padilla B, Gil JV, Manzanares P. Challenges of the non-conventional yeast *Wickerhamomyces anomalus* in winemaking. Fermentation. 2018;**4**(68):1-14. DOI: 10.3390/fermentation4030068

[113] Domizio P, House JF, Joseph CML, Bisson LF, Bamforth CW. *Lachancea thermotolerans* as an alternative yeast for the production of beer. Journal of the Institute of Brewing. 2016;**122**:599-604. DOI: 10.1002/jib.362

[114] Osburn K, Amaral J, Metcalf SR, Nickens DM, Rogers CM, Sausen C, et al. Primary souring: A novel bacteria-free method for sour beer production. Food Microbiology. 2018;**70**:76-84. DOI: 10.1016/j.fm.2017.09.007

[115] Varela J, Varela C. Microbiological strategies to produce beer and wine with reduced ethanol concentration. Current Opinion in Biotechnology. 2019;**56**:88-96. DOI: 10.1016/j.copbio.2018.10.003

[116] De Francesco G, Turchetti B, Sileoni V, Marconi O, Perretti G. Screening of new strains of *Saccharomycodes ludwigii* and *Zygosaccharomyces rouxii* to produce low-alcohol beer. Journal of the Institute of Brewing. 2015;**121**:113-121. DOI: 10.1002/jib.185

[117] De Francesco G, Sannino C, Sileoni V, Marconi O, Filippucci S, Tasselli G, et al. *Mrakia gelida* in brewing process: An innovative production of low alcohol beer using a psychrophilic yeast strain. Food Microbiology. 2018;**76**:354-362. DOI: 10.1016/j.fm.2018.06.018

[118] Saerens S, Swiegers JH. Production of low-alcohol or alcohol-free beer with *Pichia kluyveri* yeast strains. 2017. Patent number: 20170226451A1

[119] Liu S, Quek AYH. Evaluation of beer fermentation with a novel yeast *Williopsis saturnus*. Food Technology and Biotechnology. 2016;**54**(4):403-412. DOI: 10.17113/ft b.54.04.16.4440

[120] Silva CF, Schwan RF, Dias ES, Wheals AE. Microbial diversity during maturation and natural processing of coffee cherries of *Coffea arabica L*. in Brazil. International Journal of Food Microbiology. 2000;**60**(2-3):251-260. DOI: 10.1016/S0168-1605(00)00315-9

[121] Avallone S, Guyot B, Brillouet JM, Olguin E, Guiraud JP. Microbiological and biochemical study of coffee fermentation. Current Microbiology. 2001;**42**(4):252-256. DOI: 10.1007/s002840110213

[122] de Melo-Pereira GV, Soccol VT, Pandey A, Medeiros ABP, Lara JMRA, Gollo AL, et al. Isolation, selection and evaluation of yeasts for use in fermentation of coffee beans by the wet process. International Journal of Food Microbiology. 2014;**188**:60-66. DOI: 10.1016/j.ijfoodmicro.2014.07.008

[123] de Melo-Pereira GV, Neto E, Soccol VT, Medeiros ABP, Woiciechowski AL, Soccol CR. Conducting starter culture-controlled fermentations of coffee beans during on-farm wet processing: Growth, metabolic analyses and sensorial effects. Food Research International. 2015;**75**:348-356. DOI: 10.1016/j.foodres.2015.06.027

[124] Lee LW, Cheong MW, Curran P, Yu B, Liu SQ. Coffee fermentation and flavor—An intricate and delicate relationship. Food Chemistry. 2015;**185**:182-191. DOI: 10.1016/j.foodchem.2015.03.124

[125] Agate AD, Bhat JV. Role of pectinolytic yeasts in the degradation of mucilage layer of *Coffea robusta* cherries. Journal of Applied Microbiology. 1966;**14**(2):256-260

[126] Masoud W, Cesar LB, Jespersen L, Jakobsen M. Yeast involved in fermentation of *Coffea arabica* in East Africa determined by genotyping and by direct denaturing gradient gel electrophoresis. Yeast. 2004;**21**(7):549-556. DOI: 10.1002/yea.1124

[127] Silva CF, Batista LR, Abreu LM, Dias ES, Schwan RF. Succession of bacterial and fungal communities during natural coffee (*Coffea arabica*) fermentation. Food Microbiology. 2008;**25**(8):951-957. DOI: 10.1016/j.fm.2008.07.003

[128] Velmourougane K. Impact of natural fermentation on physicochemical, microbiological and cup quality characteristics of arabica and robusta coffee. Proceedings of the National Academy of Sciences, India Section B: Biological Sciences. 2013;**83**(2):233-239. DOI: 10.1007/s40011-012-0130-1

[129] Masoud W, Jespersen L. Pectin degrading enzymes in yeasts involved in fermentation of *Coffea arabica* in East Africa. International Journal of Food Microbiology. 2006;**110**(3):291-296. DOI: 10.1016/j.ijfoodmicro.2006.04.030

[130] Silva CF, Vilela DM, Souza CC, Duarte WF, Dias DR, Schwan RF. Evaluation of a potential starter culture for enhance quality of coffee fermentation. World Journal of Microbiology and Biotechnology. 2013;**29**(2):235-247. DOI: 10.1007/s11274-012-1175-2

[131] Evangelista SR, Pedrozo Miguel MGC, Cordeiro CS, Silva CF, Pinheiro ACM, Schwan RF. Inoculation of starter cultures in a semi-dry coffee (*Coffea arabica*) fermentation process. Food Microbiology. 2014;**44**:87-95. DOI: 10.1016/j.fm.2014.05.013

[132] Ardhana M, Fleet G. The microbial ecology of cocoa bean fermentations in Indonesia. International Journal of Food Microbiology. 2003;**86**(1-2):87-99. DOI: 10.1016/S0168-1605(03)00081-3

[133] Schwan RF, Wheals AE. The microbiology of cocoa fermentation and its role in chocolate quality. Critical Reviews in Food Science and Nutrition. 2004;**44**(4):205-221. DOI: 10.1080/10408690490464104

[134] Camu N, De Winter T, Verbrugghe K, Cleenwerck I, Vandamme P, Takrama JS, et al. Dynamics and biodiversity of populations of lactic acid bacteria and acetic acid bacteria involved in spontaneous heap fermentation of cocoa beans in Ghana. Applied and Environmental Microbiology. 2007;**73**(6):1809-1824. DOI: 10.1128/AEM.02189-06

[135] Lima LJR, Almeida MH, Rob Nout MJ, Zwietering MH. *Theobroma cacao* L., The food of the Gods: Quality determinants of commercial cocoa beans, with particular reference to the impact of fermentation. Critical Reviews in Food Science and Nutrition. 2011;**51**(8):731-761. DOI: 10.1080/10408391003799913

[136] Sanchez J, Guiraud JP, Gaizy P. A study of the polygalacturonase activity of several yeast strains isolated from cocoa. Applied Microbiology and Biotechnology. 1984;**20**(4):262-267. DOI: 10.1007/BF00250636

[137] Crafack M, Mikkelsen MB, Saerens S, Knudsen M, Blennow A, Lowor S, et al. Influencing cocoa flavour using *Pichia kluyveri* and *Kluyveromyces marxianus* in a defined mixed starter culture for cocoa fermentation. International Journal of Food Microbiology. 2013;**167**(1):103-116. DOI: 10.1016/j.ijfoodmicro.2013.06.024

[138] Dario A, Eskes AB. Process for the fermentation of cocoa beans to modify their aromatic profile. 2012. Patent number: EP2456321 A2

[139] Saerens S, Swiegers JH. Enhancement of cocoa quality and flavor by using pichia kluyveri yeast starter culture for cocoa fermentation. 2013. Patent number: WO2013064678 A1

[140] Turner TR, James EK, Poole PS. The plant microbiome. Genome Biology. 2013;**14**(6):209. DOI: 10.1186/gb-2013-14-6-209

[141] Schlaeppi K, Bulgarelli D. The plant microbiome at work. Molecular Plant Microbe Interactions. 2015;**28**(3):212-217. DOI: 10.1094/MPMI-10-14-0334-FI

[142] Mendes R, Garbeva P, Raaijmakers JM. The rhizosphere microbiome: Significance of plant beneficial, plant pathogenic, and human pathogenic microorganisms. FEMS Microbiology Reviews. 2013;**37**(5):634-663. DOI: 10.1111/1574-6976.12028

[143] Kaur H. Sustainable environmental biotechnology. In: Kumar R, Sharma A, Ahluwalia S, editors. Advances in Environmental Biotechnology. Singapore: Springer; 2017. pp. 145-154. DOI: 10.1007/978-981-10-4041-2_8

[144] Nassar AH, El-Tarabily KA, Sivasithamparam K. Promotion of plant

growth by an auxin-producing isolate of the yeast *Williopsis saturnus* endophytic in maize (*Zea mays* L.) roots. Biology and Fertility of Soils. 2005;**42**(2):97-108. DOI: 10.1007/s00374-005-0008-y

[145] Amprayn K, Rose MT, Kecskes M, Pereg L, Nguyen HT, Kennedy IR. Plant growth promotion characteristics of soil yeast (*Candida tropicalis* HY) and its effectiveness for promoting rice growth. Applied Soil Ecology. 2012;**61**:295-299. DOI: 10.1016/j.apsoil.2011.11.009

[146] El-Tarabily KA, Sivasithamparam A. Potential of yeasts as biocontrol agents of soil-borne fungal plant pathogens and as plant growth promoters. Mycoscience. 2006;**47**:25-35. DOI: 10.1007/s10267-005-0268-2

[147] Nutaratat P, Srisuk N, Arunrattiyakorn P, Limtong S. Plant growth-promoting traits of epyphitic and endophytic yeasts isolated from rice and sugar leaves in Thailand. Fungal Biology. 2014;**118**(8):683-694. DOI: 10.1016/j.funbio.2014.04.010

[148] Fu S-F, Sun P-F, Lu H-Y, Wei J-Y, Xiao H-S, Fang W-T, et al. Plant growth-promoting traits of yeasts isolated from the phyllosphere and rhizosphere of *Drosera spatulata* Lab. Fungal Biology. 2016;**120**(3):433-448. DOI: 10.1016/j.funbio.2015.12.006

[149] Xin G, Glawe D, Doty SL. Characterization of three endophytic, indole-3-acetic acid-producing yeasts occurring in *Populus* trees. Mycological Research. 2009;**113**:973-980. DOI: 10.1016/j.mycres.2009.06.001

[150] Khan Z, Guelich G, Phan H, Redman R, Doty S. Bacterial and yeast endophytes from poplar and willow promote growth in crop plants and grasses. ISRN Agronomy. 2012;**2012**:890280. DOI: 10.5402/2012/890280

[151] Knoth JL, Kim S-H, Ettl GJ, Doty SL. Effects of cross host species inoculation of nitrogen-fixing endophytes on growth and leaf physiology of maize. Global Change Biology Bioenergy. 2012;**5**(4):408-418. DOI: 10.1111/gcbb.12006

[152] Knoth JL, Kim S-H, Ettl GJ, Doty SL. Biological nitrogen fixation and biomass accumulation within poplar clones as a result of inoculations with endophyte consortia. New Phytologist. 2014;**201**:599-609. DOI: 10.1111/nph.12536

[153] Mukherjee S, Sen SK. Exploration of novel rhizospheric yeast isolate as fertilizing soil inoculant for improvement of maize cultivation. Journal of the Science of Food and Agriculture. 2015;**95**(7):1491-1499. DOI: 10.1002/jsfa.6848

[154] Firrincieli A, Otillar R, Salamov A, Schmutz J, Khan Z, Redman RS, et al. Genome sequence of the plant growth promoting endophytic yeast *Rhodotorula graminis* WP1. Frontiers in Microbiology. 2015;**6**:978. DOI: 10.3389/fmicb.2015.00978

[155] Ignatova LV, Brazhnikova YV, Berzhanova RZ, Mukasheva TD. Plant growth-promotion and antifungal activity of yeasts from dark chestnut soil. Microbiological Research. 2015;**175**:78-83. DOI: 10.1016/j.micres.2015.03.008

[156] Spaepen S, Vanderleyden J, Remans R. Indole-3-acetic acid in microbial and microorganism-plant signaling. FEMS Microbiology Reviews. 2007;**31**(4):425-448. DOI: 10.1111/j.1574-6976.2007.00072.x

[157] Vacheron J, Desbrosses G, Bouffaud ML, Touraine B, Moenne-Loccoz Y, Muller D, et al. Plant growth-promoting rhizobacteria and roots system functioning. Frontiers in Plant Science. 2013;**4**:356. DOI: 10.3389/fpls.2013.00356

[158] Alonso LM, Kleiner D, Ortega E. Spores of the mycorrhizal fungus *Glomus mosseae* host yeasts that solubilize phosphate and accumulate polyphosphates. Mycorrhiza. 2008;**18**:197-204. DOI: 10.1007/s00572-008-0172-7

[159] Sarabia M, Jakobsen I, Gronlund M, Carreon-Abud Y, Larsen J. Rhizosphere yeasts improve P uptake of a maize arbuscular mycorrhizal association. Applied Soil Ecology. 2017;**125**:18-25. DOI: 10.1016/j.apsoil.2017.12.012

[160] Vassileva M, Azcon R, Barea J-M, Vassilev N. Rock phosphate solubilization by free and encapsulated cells of *Yarowia lipolytica*. Process Biochemistry. 2000;**35**:693-397. DOI: 10.1016/S0032-9592(99)00132-6

[161] El-Tarabily KA. Suppression of *Rhizoctonia solani* diseases of sugar beet by antagonistic and plant growth-promoting yeasts. Journal of Applied Microbiology. 2004;**96**:69-75. DOI: 10.1046/j.1365-2672.2003.02043.x

[162] Sansone G, Rezza I, Calvente V, Benuzzi D, de Tosetti MIS. Control of *Botrytis cinerea* strains resistant to iprodione in apple with rhodotorulic acid and yeasts. Postharvest Biology and Technology. 2005;**35**:245-251. DOI: 10.1016/j.postharvbio.2004.09.005

[163] Glick BR. Bacteria with ACC deaminase can promote plant growth and help to feed the world. Microbiological Research. 2013;**169**(1):30-39. DOI: 10.1016/j.micres.2013.09.009

Section 4

Industrial Bioproducts

Chapter 6

The Oleaginous Red Yeast *Rhodotorula/Rhodosporidium*: A Factory for Industrial Bioproducts

Mathew Lyman, Salustra Urbin, Cheryl Strout and Bonnee Rubinfeld

Abstract

Rhodotorula genus, amended in 2015, is polyphyletic and contains *Rhodotorula* species that grow as single-cell yeast (monomorphic) and reproduce asexually via budding/fission (anamorphic); it also contains *Rhodosporidium* species that reproduce sexually (teleomorphic) and alternate between a yeast phase and dikaryotic filamentous phase (dimorphic). Several species of these "red yeast" produce industrial bioproducts, namely biofuel feedstocks, carotenoids, enzymes, and biosurfactants. This chapter highlights the biotechnology areas that *Rhodotorula/Rhodosporidium* contributes to and the future market value of those industries. The primary yeast species to be discussed include *Rhodosporidium toruloides, Rhodotorula glutinis, Rhodosporidium diobovatum, Rhodosporidium kratochvilovae, Rhodotorula graminis, Rhodotorula babjevae, and Rhodotorula taiwanensis.*

Keywords: *Rhodotorula*, *Rhodosporidium*, red yeast, oleaginous, carotenoids, biofuels, biodiesel, antioxidants, DAAO enzyme, PAL enzyme, PEFA, surfactants, antagonistic yeast

1. Introduction

The aim of this chapter is to discuss the *Rhodotorula* genus in the context of biotechnology; it is not meant to be an academic "deep-dive" into all things known about the topic (their discovery and classification in the early 1900s could be a separate chapter unto itself [1]). The word "oleaginous" used in the chapter title is important, and it means "oil producing" or "rich in oils." Much of the interest in these yeast stems from the fact that they often store excess carbon as triacylglycerols (TAG), not as polysaccharides [2]. These lipids can account for up to 70% of the cells dry mass depending on growth conditions, and these oils can be harvested and used as raw material in second-generation biodiesel production. Some *Rhodotorula* species also produce glycolipids, known as polyol esters of fatty acids (PEFA), which have broad interest in the biosurfactant industry. Several emerging publications and patents have been reported in this area. In addition, these yeasts are indeed "pinkish red." These hues are carotenoid compounds produced by the yeast; these natural dyes can be extracted from *Rhodotorula/Rhodosporidium* and used in the food and vitamin industries. This chapter will further expand upon these intriguing facts and illustrate other examples that are in the scientific and patent literature, all while highlighting the future market potential of these "industrious" yeast.

IntechOpen

1.1 A brief introduction to the *Rhodotorula* genus

There was a major revision of the subphylum *Pucciniomycotina* (Phylum *Basidiomycota*, Kingdom *Fungi*) published by Wang et al. in 2015; therefore, this chapter will focus solely on species that are categorized under the revised *Rhodotorula* genus in the Sporidiobolaceae family. Species to be discussed include *Rhodosporidium toruloides, Rhodotorula glutinis, Rhodosporidium diobovatum, Rhodosporidium kratochvilovae, Rhodotorula graminis, Rhodotorula babjevae, and Rhodotorula taiwanensis*. Species that were removed from the *Rhodotorula* genus in 2015, for example, *Rhodotorula bogoriensis* (reclassified as *Pseudohyphozyma bogoriensis*), will not be discussed in detail, even though it produces sophorolipid biosurfactants and is of industrial interest [3–5].

It is noteworthy that the *Rhodotorula* genus is polyphyletic. It contains *Rhodotorula* species that grow as single-cell yeast (monomorphic) and reproduce asexually via budding/fission (anamorphic) [6]. It also contains *Rhodosporidium* species that reproduce sexually (teleomorphic) and alternate between a yeast phase and dikaryotic filamentous phase (dimorphic). For *Rhodosporidium*, sexual reproduction begins with the fusing of compatible haploid yeast cells. They then grow as dikaryotic hyphae/mycelium, during which diploid teliospores are produced. Teliospores germinate forming basidium (where karyogamy and meiosis occur) and then extrude haploid basidiospores. Germination of basidiospores then restores the yeast phase of growth [7, 8]. Thus, the yeast phases of *Rhodotorula* and *Rhodosporidium* species are virtually indistinguishable. It is notable that "all known *Rhodosporidium* species [have been] isolated as haploid yeasts and have a bipolar mating behavior, i.e., their strains belong to either one of two complementary mating types, designated *A1* and *A2* or *A* and *a*" [9]. Due to this mating behavior, *Rhodosporidium toruloides* is being developed as an alternative biotechnology platform to *Saccharomyces cerevisiae* [10] with unique biochemical pathways for the production of biofuels, carotenoids, and industrial enzymes.

1.2 The industrial markets of the genus *Rhodotorula*

The most relevant question for the purposes of this chapter, regardless of the details of any given species, is "what biotechnology markets are impacted by the *Rhodotorula* genus?" **Figure 1** summarizes the five major industrial markets where *Rhodotorula* yeast is utilized (or will likely be utilized in the future). These include biofuels, carotenoids, enzyme production (e.g. D-Amino acid oxidase (DAAO) and L-Phenylalanine ammonia lyase (PAL)), biosurfactants, and antagonistic yeast.

1.2.1 Biofuels

Biofuels continue to grow as a global industry, despite the challenges in production capacity and automotive engine compatibility [11]. The biofuels market size is expected to reach USD ~218 billion by 2022 [12]. For example, United Airlines announced in 2018 that it would begin blending more biofuel with conventional fuel, with a goal to reduce greenhouse emissions by 50% on all flights by 2050. It is expected that other airlines will follow suit, further increasing biofuel demand. Thus, there continues to be a need for microbial factories to produce biofuels [13, 14], especially given the market competition of using vegetable oils in both the food and biodiesel sectors [15]. Microorganisms may contribute to biofuel production in several ways; bisabolene (a diesel alternative) can be produced through bioengineering the isoprenoid pathway [16], and alkanes and alkenes can be produced through fatty acid biosynthesis inside the cell [15, 17]. Furthermore, microbial triglycerides,

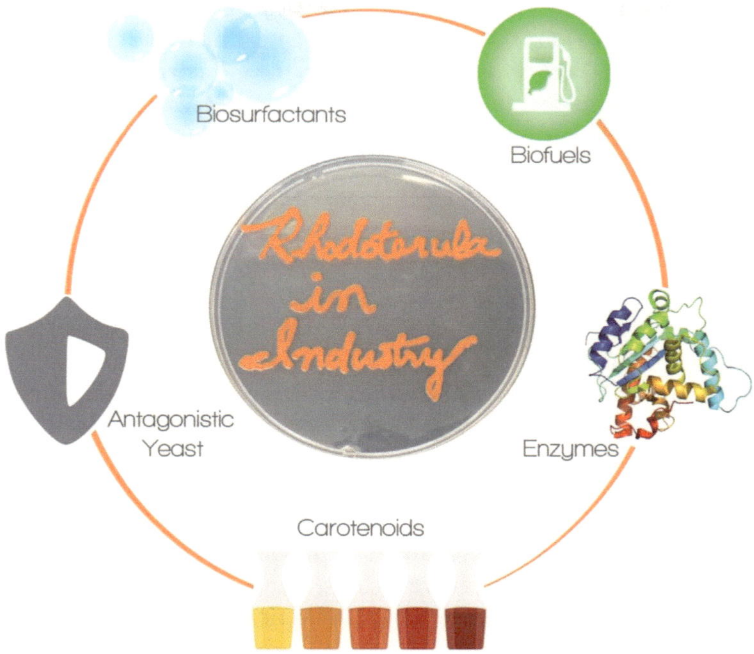

Figure 1.
The primary biotechnology industries impacted by the Rhodotorula genus. "Rhodotorula in Industry" was written in Rhodotorula taiwanensis MD1149 on a Hommel minimal salt (HMS) agar plate supplemented with glucose.

fatty acids, and other lipids can be converted to fatty acid methyl esters (FAME) by transesterification with methanol; FAME molecules are the primary component in biodiesel fuel.

The biofuels industry is largely divided between two types of fuel: biodiesel and bioethanol. These biofuels are further separated as "first generation, second generation, third generation, or fourth generation." First-generation biofuels are produced using feedstocks that can also be used for food (e.g. soy, canola, or sunflower oils). These oils are transesterified into FAME by reacting a triacylglyceride with a short alcohol—usually methanol—in the presence of a catalyst (strong base) and heat. By contrast, second-generation biofuels are produced using *non-food/non-edible* sources such as wood, organic waste, and food crop waste. Second-generation biofuels are preferred as they do not utilize food crops for fuel. Third-generation biofuels are produced by engineered algae; fourth-generation biofuels are aimed at using biomass that captures CO_2 while producing lipids that can be converted into biofuel. In this context, *Rhodotorula/Rhodosporidium* species that are used in biodiesel production are classified as "second generation" biodiesel producers that accumulate single-cell oils (SCOs); they will be discussed later in this chapter.

1.2.2 Carotenoids

In addition to lipids, these yeasts also produce carotenoids, which are of industrial interest. A recent report entitled "Global Carotenoid Market – Growth, Trends, and Forecast (2018–2023)" predicted a global carotenoid market of USD 2 billion by 2023 [18]. Carotenoids are yellow, orange, and red pigments produced by microorganisms, algae, higher plants, and some animals; these compounds are responsible for giving *Rhodotorula* species their "Red Yeast" moniker. Common examples of carotenoids include alpha-carotene, beta-carotene, beta-cryptoxanthin, lutein, lycopene, torulene, and torularhodin. Carotenoids are effective "quenchers" of reactive oxygen species (ROS), and the protective health effects of dietary carotenoids (as antioxidants) are of intense interest to the industrial research community [19]. Some carotenoids found in fruits and vegetables can be converted into vitamin A, namely beta-carotene, and to a lesser extent alpha-carotene and beta-cryptoxanthin (note: these compounds are often referred to as "provitamin A"). The impact of Vitamin A on human health is nicely summarized by Ulbricht et al. [20]. Carotenoids may also be used as natural coloring agents in the food, cosmetic, and pharmaceutical industries [21].

1.2.3 Enzymes

The *Rhodotorula/Rhodosporidium* enzymes, D-Amino acid oxidase (DAAO) and L-Phenylalanine ammonia lyase (PAL), have notable utility within industry. DAAO is a "FAD-dependent oxidoreductase that catalyzes stereospecifically the oxidative deamination of d-amino acids to α-keto acids, ammonia, and hydrogen peroxide" [22]. Even though DAAOs have been identified in a wide range of living organisms (e.g. bacteria, fungi, humans) [23], DAAO from certain *Rhodotorula* strains—discussed later in this chapter—has advantages over others, mainly due to a higher turnover rate and their increased stability of FAD binding [24]. This makes them ideal for the enzymatic deamination of cephalosporin C to 7-(5-oxoadipoamido)-cephalosporanic acid, an important intermediate for the production of cephalosporin [25]. Cephalosporin antibiotics are the largest selling class of antibiotics in a market, which is expected to reach USD 57 billion by 2024 [26, 27]. The PAL enzyme is also a major contributor to the enzymatic synthesis of "industrially relevant biomolecules," namely pure L-phenylalanine (L-Phe), L-phenylalanine methyl ester (L-PM), and para-hydroxycinnamic acid (p-HCA) [28]. L-Phe, being an essential amino acid, is used in food formulations, feed for livestock, dietary supplements, and nutraceuticals [29]. L-PM is a precursor in the production of the sweetener aspartame [28], and p-HCA has utility in the cosmetic, health, and flavoring industries [30].

1.2.4 Biosurfactants

The biosurfactant market is estimated to be worth over USD 2.7 billion by 2024, primarily driven by their usage in the personal care and cosmetic industries [31]. Biosurfactants are small molecules that contain both hydrophilic and hydrophobic moieties and reduce the surface tension between oil and water mixtures (colloquially they are known as "green detergents" or "bio-soaps"); they are produced by several microbial species, viz., bacteria, yeast, and fungi [32, 33], and they are utilized extensively in multiple industries: cosmetics, food, explosive, pharmaceutical, detergents, and paints [34, 35]. The primary market barrier for biosurfactants is the vast library of existing chemical surfactants produced from petroleum feedstocks; end users can choose from hundreds of synthetic surfactants to fulfill their industry need. A major drawback is that chemical/synthetic surfactants can accumulate in the environment and are toxic to microbes, plants, aquatic life, and higher vertebrates including humans [36]. Therefore, because biosurfactants are biodegradable and petroleum-independent, their value will likely increase as pollution increases.

1.2.5 Antagonistic yeast

Rhodotorula species also play a role in the market of biocontrol agents, also known as antagonistic yeast. Significant losses in harvested fruit occur from decay by filamentous fungi such as *Botrytis cinerea* and *Penicillium expansum* [37]. In order to replace or augment chemical fungicides, biological control agents have been studied heavily the past two decades, with some yeast-based biocontrol products commercially available for specific commodities [38]. The ability to control different rots, on different fruits/vegetables, is still an important goal when developing postharvest biocontrol products. Therefore, antagonistic yeasts continue to be an active area of research, and several *Rhodotorula* species have shown promise in this field.

2. Species utilized in biotechnology

2.1 *Rhodosporidium toruloides*

Rhodosporidium toruloides has tremendous potential as a workhorse for multiple industrial applications [39]. It can grow on a variety of carbon sources associated with modern waste streams, and its bioproducts can be used in antibiotic manufacturing, biofuel synthesis, and the food industry.

R. toruloides is a nonpathogenic, aerobic, oleaginous red yeast that has been isolated from a variety of sources, e.g. conifers, soil, wood pulp, dry leaves, and a salt farm [2]. It is able to accumulate lipids to more than 70% of its dry cell weight [40–43]; this occurs when carbon is in excess during growth, and other key nutrients such as nitrogen are sparse [44]. This lipid production can occur on a variety of different carbon sources, e.g. sugarcane juice, crude glycerol, lignocellulosic hydrolysates, vegetable market waste, and Jerusalem artichoke plants [45–49].

Due to the ability of *R. toruloides* to use different types of carbon sources for growth and lipid production, several studies have been carried out on growing this organism using "cheap" carbon sources that are the waste streams from other large industries, namely food waste and crude glycerol waste. Food wastes are an appealing nutrient source, because they are cheap, abundant, and decrease the environmental impact of disposing of these materials using traditional consumer and agricultural waste infrastructure [50, 51]. Crude glycerol is of interest as a "waste" source as the biofuel industry generates ~10% w/w of glycerol for every batch of biodiesel produced; *R. toruloides* has been shown to use crude glycerol as a carbon source for the production of microbial lipids of interest, even in the presence of impurities [52, 53]. In addition, it has been reported that *R. toruloides* has the ability to degrade/utilize hydrocarbon fuels [54]. This opens the possibility of using this yeast as a bioremediation tool for oil contaminated soil.

The bioproducts produced by *R. toruloides* are also of intense interest, namely lipids, enzymes, and carotenoids. Wild-type and engineered strains of *R. toruloides* are truly oleaginous. They produce lipids at high titer making them promising organisms for the production of lipid-based chemicals such as biofuels, lubricants, surfactants, solvents, waxes, creams, and adhesives [2, 55, 56]. It has been shown that under low nitrogen conditions, growth on simple sugars, like glucose, fructose, xylose, or the carbohydrate glycerol, can increase TAG production [55]. To this end, several groups are working to further increase lipid production using engineered strains of *R. toruloides,* primarily for biofuels [45, 56, 57]. As a practical example, scientists in Brazil have performed a successful diesel engine test using biodiesel manufactured from lipids produced by *R. toruloides* when the organism was grown in sugarcane juice (carbon source) and urea (nitrogen source) [48].

R. toruloides is also a "gold mine" for industrial enzymes. It produces a high titer of esterase enzymes, which makes this organism of immense interest to the drug industry. For example, the process of making antibiotics in the cephalosporin class of compounds requires 3-acyloxymethyl cephalosporins to be enzymatically deacylated to the more stable intermediary 3-acyloxymethyl cephalosporins. This can be achieved by the esterase enzymes produced by *R. toruloides*. Another enzyme produced by *R. toruloides* is phenylalanine ammonia-lyase (PAL), which is a major contributor to the enzymatic synthesis of pure L-phenylalanine (L-Phe), L-phenylalanine methyl ester (L-PM), and para-hydroxycinnamic acid (p-HCA) [28].

R. toruloides has also played an important role in the development of an enzyme substitution treatment of Phenylketonuria (PKU) [58, 59], a genetic mutation manifesting in the inability to metabolize L-Phe. In the human diet, L-phenylalanine is found naturally in protein foods, such as eggs, meats, fish, cheese, and soybeans, and is also produced as a product that can be added to foods, in the case of aspartame. The buildup of L-Phe in the blood is extremely toxic and impacts neurological function in the form of seizures, tremors, and loss of muscle coordination, especially in the extremities [58]. Newborns are screened for PKU at birth to increase the chances of early discovery and attempt to limit the effects of PKU. A new drug, Palynziq™, was developed based on some of the research that involved *R. toruloides* along with other PAL producing species; it was approved by the FDA in May 2018 as an enzyme substitution therapy for PKU [59].

2.2 *Rhodotorula glutinis*

Rhodotorula glutinis, like *R. toruloides*, is of high industrial importance as it also synthesizes numerous valuable compounds: lipids (SCO, single-cell oils), enzymes (in particular, PAL), and carotenoids (lycopene, β-carotene, torulene, and torularhodin). An example workflow of harvesting these bioproducts from these species is shown in **Figure 2**.

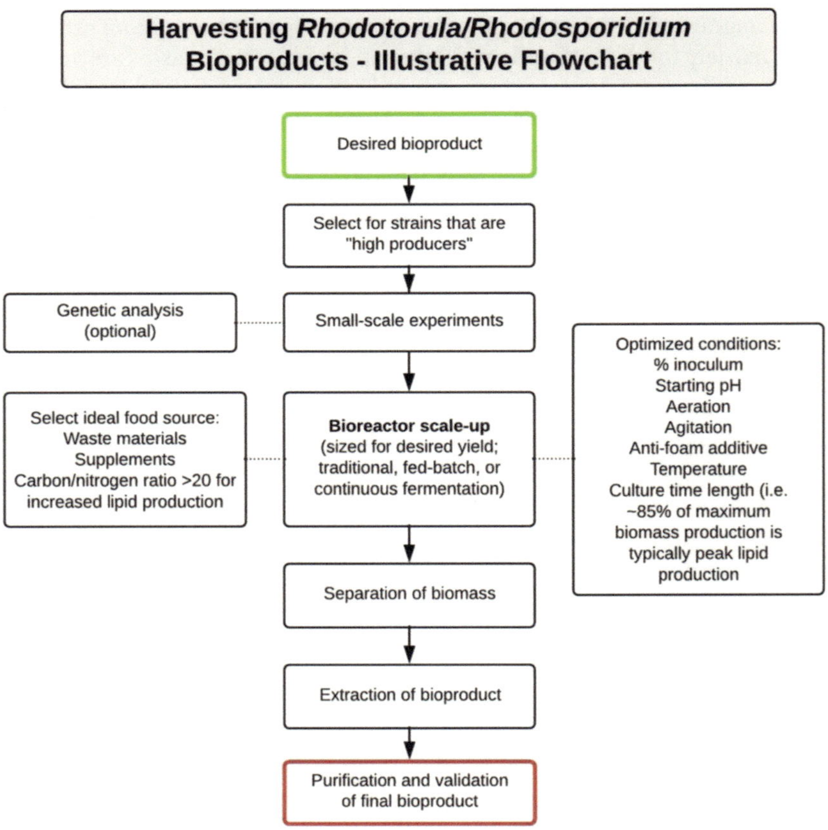

Figure 2.
An example workflow of harvesting bioproducts from members of the Rhodotorula genus.

R. glutinis isolates have been isolated from air, fruit, seawater, soil, grass, milk, and cheese products [60, 61]. Previously, 370 collection strains were assigned to this species based upon color and growth properties; however, additional methods—namely genetic sequencing—have pared this list to a few dozen strains [61]. The majority of these strains are spherical, ellipsoidal, or elongated in shape; aerobic; and mesophilic, although some can thrive under lower temperatures. They use different sources of carbon for growth: glucose, galactose, sucrose, maltose, trehalose, ethanol, glycerol, and hexadecane. *R. glutinis* lack the capacity to perform sugar fermentation and can grow in salt (10% NaCl) but cannot tolerate high sugar (>50% glucose). Depending on strain and growth conditions, their colonies are smooth, moist, and mucoid. As with most species in the *Rhodotorula* genus, color can be creamy, yellow, salmon, pink, orange coral, and blood red due to the production of carotenoids [60].

R. glutinis strains also produce several microbial oils—dominated by oleic, linoleic, palmitic, and stearic acid [62, 63], and the lipid content in their biomass can reach up to 72% [64]. Numerous factors can affect the lipid content and distribution including choice of strain, carbon sources (molasses, glucose, sucrose, glycerol, or waste materials), nitrogen sources (ammonium sulfate or chloride, yeast extract, or monosodium glutamate wastewater), C/N ratio, and cultivation times. These factors result in a wide lipid content distribution between 18 and 66% [60]. Additionally, investigators have worked to increase microbial oil production by either improving culture medium (Chinese patent CN102559788A) or by genetically engineering *R. glutinis* (Chinese patent CN102796675B).

It is noteworthy that several conditions were evaluated for the co-production of both lipid and carotenoids; variables tested included irradiation (as a stressor), temperatures, and C/N ratios. This allowed for the development of a two-stage cultivation strategy where the first stage maximized biomass and carotenoid production under irradiation/high temperature and then maximized lipid content when switched to dark/low temperature [63]. Additional growth studies have evaluated the effect of pH with potato wastewater and glycerol [65], modulating air flow rates using glycerol with yeast extract as the nutrient supply without pH control [66] and using lignocellulosic biomass [67]. Other parameters for scale-up were explored using an airlift bioreactor with mixed carbon sources [68]. *R. glutinis* has also been genetically engineered by introducing both the beta-carotene biosynthesis genes and cellulase genes to increase yields and co-production [69].

Per other industrial applications, *R. glutinis* has been evaluated as a biocontrol agent for post-harvest microbial diseases of fruit (US patent US5525132A). To this end, it has been shown to significantly reduce the incidence of the gray mold, *Botrytis cinerea* on strawberries and apples [70, 71] possibly due to the attachment capability of the antagonistic *R. glutinis* to *B. cinerea* [72]. *R. glutinis* was also used in combination with rhamnolipids to be more efficacious against *Alternaria alternata* infection in cherry tomato fruit than either agent alone [73].

It is also interesting that *R. glutinis* has been isolated during the production of olive oil and during the fermentation and storage of green and black olives in the USA [74, 75]. Olive processing results in the generation of large quantities of olive mill wastewater (OMW) high in phenol. Advantageously, *R. glutinis* has been utilized to treat OMW by dephenolization [76].

2.3 *Rhodosporidium diobovatum*

Rhodosporidium diobovatum has been identified as being a top-tier lipid producer among a group of 69 varied oleaginous yeast strains when glucose is used as the sole carbon source; it is also amenable to scalability [77, 78]. However, biofuel research has also focused on *R. diobovatum* as a second-generation biodiesel producer due to its ability to consume the impure glycerol waste that is created as a byproduct of first-generation biodiesel production [77]. For example, it was recently reported that *R. diobovatum* could be an "effective strain for production of neutral lipids" given its high yields of oleic, palmitic, and linoleic acid [79], although growth on glucose produced more TAGs than glycerol. Importantly, a glycerol consumption strategy would allow for the continued use and optimization of the first-generation biodiesel production pipelines, while simultaneously allowing investment in the development of second-generation approaches.

Interestingly, it has been reported that up to 70% of the cost to make biodiesel could be accrued *after* the production of the cell biomass, when chemical methods of extracting TAGs are used [80]. This is a costly process that requires the complete drying of biomass, full chemical diffusion of solvent into the cells [81], yeast cell wall disruption, and lipid extraction [2]. The *direct* conversion of wet biomass to biodiesel is the ideal solution, but current methods for that are not scalable, require high temperatures, have lengthy reaction periods, or utilize expensive catalysts [82]. Recent advances with microalgae utilized an ionic liquid for wet cell disruption and lipid extraction in less than 1.5 hours [83]. This same method was effective for *R. diobovatum* and was optimized to produce 97.1% conversion of maximum FAME yields in 2.5 hours at 65°C. They did note a loss of ~40% of their KOH catalyst but conclude that switching from a homogenous to a heterogeneous catalyst could mitigate this [80]. Therefore, research is ongoing to develop *R. diobovatum* as top biofuel production species.

R. diobovatum is also being examined in several novel applications. These include as a way to produce the vitamin supplement glutathione (GSH) [84], which has reported antioxidant properties, and also can be utilized as an anti-toxicant, as a cell metabolism modulator, and potentially as a neuromediator [85]. GSH is synthesized by canonical yeasts but was found in *R. diobovatum* using high performance liquid chromatography (HPLC). Consequently, the *R. diobovatum* synthase genes have been identified and characterized, with the expectation that it could be a valuable industrial producer of GSH in future [84]. This species also has potential as a bioremediation agent for fertilizer pollution. It efficiently assimilates nitrogen at higher rates than other yeasts and may become a useful tool for treating agriculture wastewater [86].

2.4 *Rhodosporidium kratochvilovae* and *Rhodotorula graminis*

Rhodosporidium kratochvilovae cultures have been used to create single-cell oil biodiesel when cultured on cane molasses, a sugar refinery waste product [87]. This biodiesel meets standard specifications in Europe and the USA for quality and purity (ASTM D6751, EN14214). The strain was originally discovered in a screen for oleaginous yeasts in Ethiopia. Of the 340 yeast isolates screened, 18 tested positive for oil production, and a *R. kratochvilovae* strain was one of three chosen as best candidates for further optimization based on productivity [88]. Multiple parameters of its cultivation were optimized for lipid production [89] prior to being used to create SCO.

Rhodotorula graminis has also been developed for biodiesel using crude glycerol and undetoxified lignocellulosic hydrolysate (hydrolyzed corn stover; aka, the stalks, leaves, and cobs that remain in fields after harvest) [90]. This strain produced a high lipid content (34% w/w) on hydrolysate and increased this production on waste crude glycerol (54% w/w) [90]. Further optimization of this production pipeline was discussed in patent US9322038B2 granted in 2016 to Washington State University for "Simultaneous saccharification and fermentation (SSF) of lignocellulosic biomass for single-cell oil production by oleaginous microorganisms," with details of strains and culture conditions therein.

R. kratochvilovae and *R. graminis* also produce carotenoids (specifically beta-carotene, torularhodin, and torulene) in order to mitigate cellular damage done by ROS [91]. The benefits of beta-carotene have been understood for some time (antioxidant), but those of torularhodin and torulene only been elucidated recently, namely their potent anti-cancer [92] and anti-microbial activity [93]. Importantly, *R. graminis* and other *Rhodotorula* species have the ability to produce these rare carotenoids at high levels [94] and represent viable options for industrial production of these compounds.

R. kratochvilovae and *R. graminis* are also involved in the biological control of plant pathogens [95]. In a screen for yeasts that control pathogenic fungal strains, *R. kratochvilovae* LS11 was found to have high antagonistic activity [96]. Further development of this strain is hoped to be achieved, and its detoxification pathways are currently being examined in detail [97]. *R. graminis* was also been examined for this application, alone and in combination with fungicide [98].

The PAL enzyme of *R. graminis* (RgrPAL) has industrial interest as it is highly stable in comparison to that of other species, and the organism has flexible culturing requirements. Mutagenesis was employed to create mutants that expressed higher levels of PAL, including an isolate that showed a fourfold increase in production [99]. RgrPAL is also useful to pharmaceutical production, as it accepts analogues of its substrate L-Phe, which can be included in peptidomimetic drugs. The enzymatic activity of RgrPAL was recently increased 28-fold using directed evolution methodology in a recent study [100].

2.5 *Rhodotorula babjevae* and *Rhodotorula taiwanensis*

It was recently published that strains of *Rhodotorula babjevae*, and other *Rhodotorula* species, produce polyol esters of fatty acids (PEFA) [101, 102], similar in composition to extracellular glycolipids reported in the 1960s [103]. The authors stated that "discovery of these PEFA-secreting yeasts may aid in improving production of renewable, sustainable, environmentally friendly surfactants for use in household and industrial cleaning products, as well as many other applications" [102]. To this end, a full patent application was submitted in 2017 by the University of California for "Methods of producing polyol lipids," with details of *Rhodotorula* strains and culture conditions that optimize PEFA production (WO2017184884A1).

It is important to note that the general utility of surfactants in industry—whether they be chemical surfactants or biosurfactants—is determined by their hydrophilic-lipophilic balance (HLB). The HLB concept was first published in 1948 brochure by Atlas Powder Company, along with a follow-up journal paper by William Griffin (an Atlas chemist) [104]. Griffin described HLB as follows: "emulsifiers consist of a molecule that combines both hydrophilic and lipophilic groups and the balance of the size and strength of these two opposite groups is called HLB. For the purpose of convenience, the effective balance of these groups is assigned a numeric value [105]." Griffin then went on to develop the HLB number system, on a scale 0–20, based on polyoxyethylene (POE)-type surfactants. Although the correct classification of surfactants in the HLB system is still being refined and debated [104, 106, 107], the concept of different surfactants having different HLB values remains the benchmark for surfactant science. An example of different surfactant HLB values, their solubility, applications, and use in industry is provided in **Table 1**.

Perhaps the greatest market barrier that biosurfactants face is their limited coverage of the HLB scale. Therefore, they can only be used in very targeted commercial applications. By contrast, hundreds of petroleum-derived chemical surfactants

Surfactant HLB	Solubility	Applications	Industry examples
1.5–3	Oil soluble	Antifoaming agents (defoamers)	Hydraulics, paper, oil drilling, machine tools
3–6	Oil soluble	Water-in-oil emulsions	Cosmetics, sunscreen, margarine
7–9	Oil soluble	Wetting and spreading agents	Herbicides, fertilizers
12–16	Water soluble	Oil-in-water-emulsions	Mayonnaise, cosmetics, dispersants
13–15	Water soluble	Detergents	Laundry and dishwashing detergents
15–18	Water soluble	Solubilizing agents	Pharmaceuticals

Table 1.
The hydrophilic-lipophilic balance (HLB) scale covers 0–20, with different industrial applications depending on the HLB value.

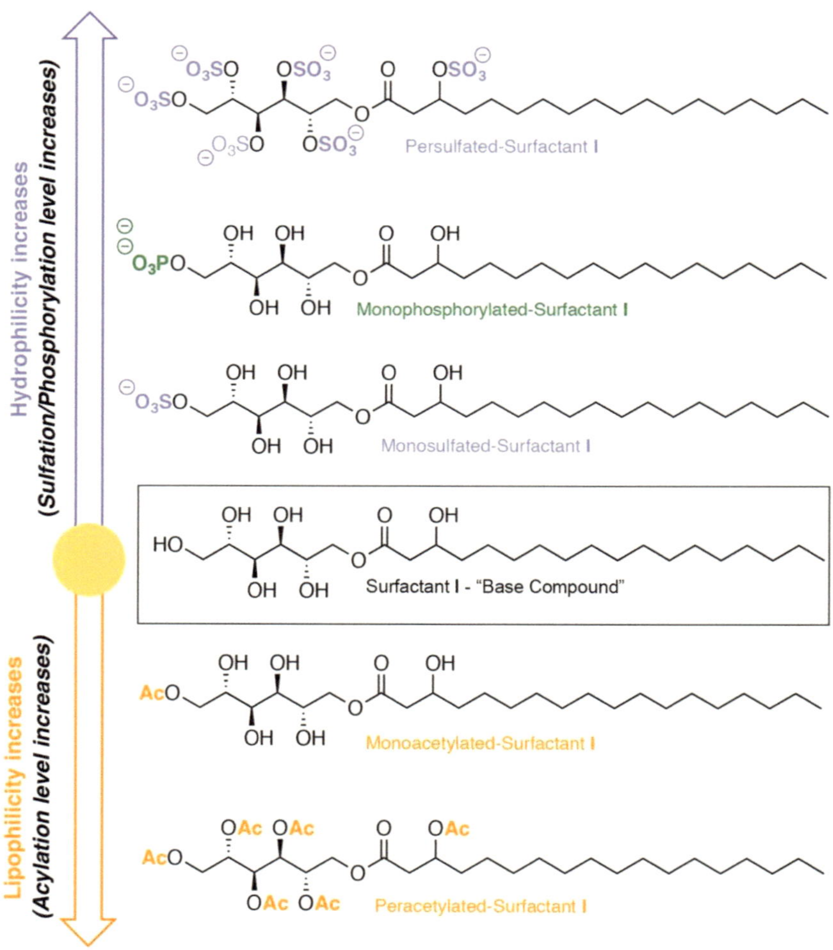

Figure 3.
A "tunable" PEFA biosurfactant. Rhodotorula taiwanensis would be genetically engineered to produce a single PEFA "base compound" and then be systematically modified to move up and down the HLB scale.

conveniently cover the entire HLB scale, to such an extent that their massive usage is now poisoning the environment [36]. Biosurfactants offer a more environmentally friendly option (biodegradable and petroleum-independent); however, there are a limited number of commercially available biosurfactants, and each one covers only a small portion of the HLB scale.

Therefore, in order to expand PEFA coverage on the HLB scale, it was recently published that a new strain of *Rhodotorula taiwanensis* produced hypoacetylated PEFA compounds compared to those produced by *Rhodotorula babjevae* [108, 109]; the difference in their acetylation profiles resulted in different surface tension of the growth medium, i.e. a different hydrophilic-lipophilic balance. It was noted in a subsequent patent filing that although the current *Rhodotorula taiwanensis* strain produced a complex mixture of acetylated and non-acetylated biosurfactants, it could be genetically engineered to produce an unmodified (non-acetylated) "base compound." This base compound could then be "tuned" to produce the full range of biosurfactants that could more extensively cover the HLB scale (**Figure 3**).

This "tunable" biosurfactant approach, using a single species of PEFA compound that can be systematically modified, provides a viable option for competing directly with all types of chemical surfactants, across all market sectors. The biosurfactant's chemical topology, highlighted by the carbohydrate unit's hydroxyl groups, offers further opportunity for chemical modifications that have a direct impact on the physical properties of the surfactant (e.g. antifoaming, emulsifying, wetting, detergent, and solubilizing). Each hydroxyl (OH) group on the molecule has the ability to be acetylated, sulfated, or phosphorylated, leading to modified versions of the parent molecule with different physicochemical properties. Therefore, modification of the hydroxyl groups by chemical and/or biochemical means will enable scientists to produce various biosurfactant products best suited for their unique industrial applications—serving markets not currently served by existing biosurfactants.

3. Conclusions

The *Rhodotorula* genus currently plays a significant role in yeast biotechnology and is poised to expand into various industrial markets: biofuels, carotenoids, biocontrol agents, enzymes, bioremediation, cosmetics, and others. Several advanced genetic systems are currently being developed for these red yeast, and they will likely become an alternative biotechnology platform to *Saccharomyces cerevisiae* [10]. The future looks bright (red) for these fascinating, diverse, and versatile oleaginous microbes.

Acknowledgements

This work was performed under the auspices of the U.S. Department of Energy by Lawrence Livermore National Laboratory under Contract DE-AC52-07NA27344. We thank Kristin Lyman for assistance with the graphic design.

Conflict of interest

The authors declare no conflict of interest.

Author details

Mathew Lyman*, Salustra Urbin, Cheryl Strout and Bonnee Rubinfeld
Biosciences and Biotechnology Division, Lawrence Livermore National Laboratory, Livermore, California, USA

*Address all correspondence to: lyman2@llnl.gov

References

[1] Hasegawa T, Banno I, Yamauchi S. A taxonomic study on the genus Rhodotorula. The Journal of General and Applied Microbiology. 1960;**6**(3):196-215

[2] Ageitos JM, Vallejo JA, Veiga-Crespo P, Villa TG. Oily yeasts as oleaginous cell factories. Applied Microbiology and Biotechnology. 2011;**90**(4):1219-1227

[3] Nunez A, Ashby R, Foglia TA, Solaiman DK. LC/MS analysis and lipase modification of the sophorolipids produced by Rhodotorula bogoriensis. Biotechnology Letters. 2004;**26**(13):1087-1093

[4] Ribeiro IA, Bronze MR, Castro MF, Ribeiro MH. Design of selective production of sophorolipids by Rhodotorula bogoriensis through nutritional requirements. Journal of Molecular Recognition: JMR. 2012;**25**(11):630-640

[5] Solaiman DK, Ashby RD, Crocker NV. High-titer production and strong antimicrobial activity of sophorolipids from Rhodotorula bogoriensis. Biotechnology Progress. 2015;**31**(4):867-874

[6] Morrow CA, Fraser JA. Sexual reproduction and dimorphism in the pathogenic basidiomycetes. FEMS Yeast Research. 2009;**9**(2):161-177

[7] Boekhout T, Fonseca Á, Sampaio JP, Bandoni RJ, Fell JW, Kwon-Chung KJ. Discussion of teleomorphic and anamorphic basidiomycetous yeasts. In: The Yeasts: A Taxonomic Study. London, UK: Elsevier; 2011

[8] Fell JW, Boekhout T, Fonseca A, Sampaio JP. Basidiomycetous yeasts. In: DJ ML, EJ ML, Lemke P, editors. The Mycota VII Part B. Systematics and Evolution. Berlin, Heidelberg: Springer-Verlag; 2001

[9] Coelho MA, Rosa A, Rodrigues N, Fonseca A, Goncalves P. Identification of mating type genes in the bipolar basidiomycetous yeast Rhodosporidium toruloides: First insight into the MAT locus structure of the Sporidiobolales. Eukaryotic Cell. 2008;**7**(6):1053-1061

[10] Kumar S, Kushwaha H, Bachhawat AK, Raghava GP, Ganesan K. Genome sequence of the oleaginous red yeast Rhodosporidium toruloides MTCC 457. Eukaryotic Cell. 2012;**11**(8):1083-1084

[11] Hassan MK, A. An overview of biofuel as a renewable energy source: Development and challenges. Procedia Engineering. 2013;**56**:39-53

[12] Research ZM. Biofuels market analysis by type (bioethanol, biodiesel), and by form (solid, liquid, and gaseous)—Global industry perspective, comprehensive analysis, and forecast, 2016-2022. 2018. https://www.zionmarketresearch.com/news/biofuels-market

[13] Lee SY, Kim HM, Cheon S. Metabolic engineering for the production of hydrocarbon fuels. Current Opinion in Biotechnology. 2015;**33**:15-22

[14] Peralta-Yahya PP, Zhang F, del Cardayre SB, Keasling JD. Microbial engineering for the production of advanced biofuels. Nature. 2012;**488**(7411):320-328

[15] Zhou Y, Eduard K, Nielsen J. Barriers and opportunities in bio-based production of hydrocarbons. Nature Energy. 2018;**3**:925-935

[16] Peralta-Yahya PP, Ouellet M, Chan R, Mukhopadhyay A, Keasling JD, Lee TS. Identification and microbial production of a terpene-based advanced biofuel. Nature Communications. 2011;**2**:483

[17] Pfleger BF, Gossing M, Nielsen J. Metabolic engineering strategies for

microbial synthesis of oleochemicals. Metabolic Engineering. 2015;**29**:1-11

[18] Intelligence Mordor. Global Carotenoid Market—Growth, Trends, and Forecast (2018-2023). 2018

[19] Fiedor J, Burda K. Potential role of carotenoids as antioxidants in human health and disease. Nutrients. 2014;**6**(2):466-488

[20] Ulbricht C, Basch E, Chao W, Conquer J, Costa D, Culwell S, et al. An evidence-based systematic review of vitamin A by the natural standard research collaboration. Journal of Dietary Supplements. 2012;**9**(4):299-416

[21] Mortensen A. Carotenoids and other pigments as natural colorants. Pure and Applied Chemistry. 2006;**78**(8):1477-1491

[22] Liu Y, Koh CMJ, Ngoh ST, Ji L. Engineering an efficient and tight D-amino acid-inducible gene expression system in Rhodosporidium/Rhodotorula species. Microbial Cell Factories. 2015;**14**:170

[23] Pollegioni L, Piubelli L, Sacchi S, Pilone MS, Molla G. Physiological functions of D-amino acid oxidases: From yeast to humans. Cellular and Molecular Life Sciences. 2007;**64**(11):1373-1394

[24] Pilone MS. D-amino acid oxidase: New findings. Cellular and Molecular Life Sciences. 2000;**57**(12):1732-1747

[25] Hsieh HC, Kuan IC, Lee SL, Tien GY, Wang YJ, Yu CY. Stabilization of D-amino acid oxidase from Rhodosporidium toruloides by immobilization onto magnetic nanoparticles. Biotechnology Letters. 2009;**31**(4):557-563

[26] Hamad B. The antibiotics market. Nature Reviews. Drug Discovery. 2010;**9**(9):675-676

[27] Research GV. Antibiotics Market Size To Reach $57.0 Billion By 2024. 2016

[28] MacDonald MC, Arivalagan P, Barre DE, MacInnis JA, D'Cunha GB. Rhodotorula glutinis phenylalanine/tyrosine ammonia lyase enzyme catalyzed synthesis of the methyl ester of Para-hydroxycinnamic acid and its potential antibacterial activity. Frontiers in Microbiology. 2016;**7**:281

[29] Ding D, Liu Y, Xu Y, Zheng P, Li H, Zhang D, et al. Improving the production of L-phenylalanine by identifying key enzymes through multi-enzyme reaction system in vitro. Scientific Reports. 2016;**6**:32208

[30] Vargas-Tah A, Gosset G. Production of cinnamic and p-Hydroxycinnamic acids in engineered microbes. Frontiers in Bioengineering and Biotechnology. 2015;**3**:116

[31] Global Market Insights I. Biosurfactants Market worth over $2.7 bn by 2024. 2018

[32] Satpute SK, Banpurkar AG, Dhakephalkar PK, Banat IM, Chopade BA. Methods for investigating biosurfactants and bioemulsifiers: A review. Critical Reviews in Biotechnology. 2010;**30**(2):127-144

[33] Uzoigwe C, Burgess JG, Ennis CJ, Rahman PK. Bioemulsifiers are not biosurfactants and require different screening approaches. Frontiers in Microbiology. 2015;**6**:245

[34] Reis RS, Pacheco GJ, Pereira AG, Freire DMG. Biosurfactants: Production and applications. In: Rosenkranz RCF, editor. Biodegradation—Life of Science. Rijeka: InTech; 2013

[35] Varvaresou A, Iakovou K. Biosurfactants in cosmetics and biopharmaceuticals. Letters in Applied Microbiology. 2015;**61**(3):214-223

[36] Rebello S, Asok AK, Mundayoor S, Jisha MS. Surfactants: Chemistry, toxicity and remediation. In: Lichtfouse E et al., editors. Pollutant Diseases, Remediation and Recycling. Switzerland: Springer International Publishing; 2013

[37] Castoria R, Filipo DC, Lima G, De Cicco V. β-1,3-glucanase activity of two saprophytic yeasts and possible mode of action as biocontrol agents against postharvest diseases. Postharvest Biology and Technology. 1997;**12**(3):293-300

[38] Liu J, Sui Y, Wisniewski M, Droby S, Liu Y. Review: Utilization of antagonistic yeasts to manage postharvest fungal diseases of fruit. International Journal of Food Microbiology. 2013;**167**(2):153-160

[39] Park YK, Nicaud JM, Ledesma-Amaro R. The engineering potential of Rhodosporidium toruloides as a workhorse for biotechnological applications. Trends in Biotechnology. 2018;**36**(3):304-317

[40] Li Q, Du W, Liu D. Perspectives of microbial oils for biodiesel production. Applied Microbiology and Biotechnology. 2008;**80**(5):749-756

[41] Singh G, Jawed A, Paul D, Bandyopadhyay KK, Kumari A, Haque S. Concomitant production of lipids and carotenoids in Rhodosporidium toruloides under osmotic stress using response surface methodology. Frontiers in Microbiology. 2016;7:1686

[42] Zhu Z, Zhang S, Liu H, Shen H, Lin X, Yang F, et al. A multi-omic map of the lipid-producing yeast Rhodosporidium toruloides. Nature Communications. 2012;**3**:1112

[43] Li Y, Zhao Z, Bai F. High-density cultivation of oleaginous yeast Rhodosporidium toruloides Y4 in fed-batch culture. Enzyme and Microbial Technology. 2007;**41**:312-317

[44] Papanikolaou S, Aggelis G. Lipids of oleaginous yeasts. Part I: Biochemistry of single cell oil production. European Journal of Lipid Science and Technology. 2011;**113**:1031-1051

[45] Fei Q, O'Brien M, Nelson R, Chen X, Lowell A, Dowe N. Enhanced lipid production by Rhodosporidium toruloides using different fed-batch feeding strategies with lignocellulosic hydrolysate as the sole carbon source. Biotechnology for Biofuels. 2016;**9**:130

[46] Hu C, Zhao X, Zhao J, Wu S, Zhao ZK. Effects of biomass hydrolysis by-products on oleaginous yeast Rhodosporidium toruloides. Bioresource Technology. 2009;**100**(20):4843-4847

[47] Singh G, Sinha S, Bandyopadhyay KK, Lawrence M, Paul D. Triauxic growth of an oleaginous red yeast Rhodosporidium toruloides on waste 'extract' for enhanced and concomitant lipid and beta-carotene production. Microbial Cell Factories. 2018;**17**(1):182

[48] Soccol CR, Dalmas Neto CJ, Soccol VT, Sydney EB, da Costa ESF, Medeiros ABP, et al. Pilot scale biodiesel production from microbial oil of Rhodosporidium toruloides DEBB 5533 using sugarcane juice: Performance in diesel engine and preliminary economic study. Bioresource Technology. 2017;**223**:259-268

[49] Zhao X, Wu S, Hu C, Wang Q, Hua Y, Zhao ZK. Lipid production from Jerusalem artichoke by Rhodosporidium toruloides Y4. Journal of Industrial Microbiology & Biotechnology. 2010;**37**(6):581-585

[50] Pham TP, Kaushik R, Parshetti GK, Mahmood R, Balasubramanian R. Food waste-to-energy conversion technologies: Current status and future directions. Waste Management. 2015;**38**:399-408

[51] Zeng Y, Xie T, Li P, Jian B, Li X, Xie Y, et al. Enhanced lipid production and nutrient utilization of food waste hydrolysate by mixed culture of oleaginous yeast Rhodosporidium toruloides and oleaginous microalgae Chlorella vulgaris. Renewable Energy. 2018;**126**:915-923

[52] Uprety BK, Swaroop Dalli S, Rakshit S. Bioconversion of crude glycerol to microbial lipid using a robust oleaginous yeast Rhodosporidium toruloides ATCC 10788 capable of growing in the presence of impurities. Energy Conversion and Management. 2017;**135**:117-128

[53] Xu J, Xuebing Z, Wang W, Du W, Liu D. Microbial conversion of biodiesel byproduct glycerol to triacylglycerols by oleaginous yeast Rhodosporidium toruloides and the individual effect of some impurities on lipid production. Biochemical Engineering Journal. 2012;**65**:30-36

[54] Kumari M, Jayanthi A. Biodegradation of diesel oil using yeast Rhodosporidium toruloides. Research Journal of Environmental Toxicology. 2011;**5**(6):369-377

[55] Zhang S, Ito M, Skerker JM, Arkin AP, Rao CV. Metabolic engineering of the oleaginous yeast Rhodosporidium toruloides IFO0880 for lipid overproduction during high-density fermentation. Applied Microbiology and Biotechnology. 2016;**100**(21):9393-9405

[56] Zhang S, Skerker JM, Rutter CD, Maurer MJ, Arkin AP, Rao CV. Engineering Rhodosporidium toruloides for increased lipid production. Biotechnology and Bioengineering. 2016;**113**(5):1056-1066

[57] Yaegashi J, Kirby J, Ito M, Sun J, Dutta T, Mirsiaghi M, et al. Rhodosporidium toruloides: A new platform organism for conversion of lignocellulose into terpene biofuels and bioproducts. Biotechnology for Biofuels. 2017;**10**:241

[58] Gamez A, Sarkissian CN, Wang L, Kim W, Straub M, Patch MG, et al. Development of pegylated forms of recombinant Rhodosporidium toruloides phenylalanine ammonia-lyase for the treatment of classical phenylketonuria. Molecular Therapy. 2005;**11**(6):986-989

[59] Levy HL, Sarkissian CN, Scriver CR. Phenylalanine ammonia lyase (PAL): From discovery to enzyme substitution therapy for phenylketonuria. Molecular Genetics and Metabolism. 2018;**124**(4):223-229

[60] Kot AM, Blazejak S, Kurcz A, Gientka I, Kieliszek M. Rhodotorula glutinis-potential source of lipids, carotenoids, and enzymes for use in industries. Applied Microbiology and Biotechnology. 2016;**100**(14):6103-6117

[61] Sampaio J. Rhodotorula Harrison. In: Kurtzman C, editor. The Yeasts: A Taxonomic Study. Amsterdam: Elsevier; 1928

[62] Easterling ER, French WT, Hernandez R, Licha M. The effect of glycerol as a sole and secondary substrate on the growth and fatty acid composition of Rhodotorula glutinis. Bioresource Technology. 2009;**100**(1):356-361

[63] Zhang Z, Zhang X, Tan T. Lipid and carotenoid production by Rhodotorula glutinis under irradiation/high-temperature and dark/low-temperature cultivation. Bioresource Technology. 2014;**157**:149-153

[64] Meng XY, Jianming Y, Xu X, Zhang L, Nie Q, Xian M. Biodiesel production from oleaginous microorganisms. Renewable Energy. 2009;**34**:1-5

[65] Kot AM, Błażejak S, Kurez A, Gientka I, Bzducha-Wrobel A, Maliszewska M, et al. Effect of initial pH of medium with potato wastewater and glycerol on protein, lipid and carotenoid biosynthesis by *Rhodotorula glutinis*. Electronic Journal of Biotechnology. 2017;**27**:25-31

[66] Karamerou EE, Theodoropoulos C, Webb C. A biorefinery approach to microbial oil production from glycerol by Rhodotorula glutinis. Biomass and Bioenergy. 2016;**89**:113-122

[67] Dai C-C, Jie T, Xie F, Dai Y-J, Zhao M. Biodiesel generation from oleaginous yeast Rhodotorula glutinis with xylose assimilating capacity. African Journal of Biotechnology. 2007;**6**(18):2130-2134

[68] Yen H-W, Chang J-T, Chang J-S. The growth of oleaginous Rhodotorula glutinis in an internal-loop airlift bioreactor by using mixture substrates of rice straw hydrolysate and crude glycerol. Biomass and Bioenergy. 2015;**80**:38-43

[69] Pi HW, Anandharaj M, Kao YY, Lin YJ, Chang JJ, Li WH. Engineering the oleaginous red yeast Rhodotorula glutinis for simultaneous beta-carotene and cellulase production. Scientific Reports. 2018;**8**(1):10850

[70] Zhang H, Wang L, Dong Y, Jiang S, Cao J, Meng R. Postharvest biological control of gray mold decay of strawberry with *Rhodotorula glutinis*. Biological Control. 2007;**40**:287-292

[71] Zhang H, Wang L, Ma L, Dong Y, Jiang S, Xu B, et al. Biocontrol of major postharvest pathogens on apple using Rhodotorula glutinis and its effects on postharvest quality parameters. Biological Control. 2009;**48**:79-83

[72] Li B, Peng H, Tian S. Attachment capability of antagonistic yeast Rhodotorula glutinis to Botrytis cinerea contributes to biocontrol efficacy. Frontiers in Microbiology. 2016;**7**:601

[73] Yan F, Xu S, Chen Y, Zheng X. Effect of rhamnolipids on Rhodotorula glutinis biocontrol of Alternaria alternate infection in cherry tomato fruit. Postharvest Biology and Technology. 2014;**97**:32-35

[74] Arroyo-Lopez FN, Querol A, Bautista-Gallego J, Garrido-Fernandez A. Role of yeasts in table olive production. International Journal of Food Microbiology. 2008;**128**(2):189-196

[75] Yousuf A, Sannino F, Addorisio V, Pirozzi D. Microbial conversion of olive oil mill wastewaters into lipids suitable for biodiesel production. Journal of Agricultural and Food Chemistry. 2010;**58**(15):8630-8635

[76] Gaye B, Takaç S. Parameters and kinetics of olive mill wastewater dephenolization by immobilized Rhodotorula glutinis cells. Environmental Technology. 2014;**35**:3074-3081

[77] Munch G. Characterization and Comparison of Different Oleaginous Yeasts and Scale-Up of Single-Cell Oil Production Using *Rhodosporidium diobovatum*. University of Manitoba; 2015

[78] Sitepu IR, Sestric R, Ignatia L, Levin D, German JB, Gillies LA, et al. Manipulation of culture conditions alters lipid content and fatty acid profiles of a wide variety of known and new oleaginous yeast species. Bioresource Technology. 2013;**144**:360-369

[79] Nasirian N, Mirzaie M, Cicek N, Levin DB. Lipid and carotenoid synthesis by Rhodosporidium diobovatum, grown on glucose versus glycerol, and its biodiesel properties. Canadian Journal of Microbiology. 2018;**64**(4):277-289

[80] Ward V, Garret M, Cicek N, Rehmann L. Direct conversion of the

oleaginous yeast Rhodosporidium diobovatum to biodiesel using the ionic liquid. ACS Sustainable Chemistry & Engineering. 2017;**5**:5562-5570

[81] Halim R, Gladman B, Danquah MK, Webley P. Oil extraction from microalgae for biodiesel production. Bioresource Technology. 2011;**102**(1):178-185

[82] Griffiths MJ, van Hille RP, Harrison ST. Selection of direct transesterification as the preferred method for assay of fatty acid content of microalgae. Lipids. 2010;**45**(11):1053-1060

[83] VCA O, Plechkova NV, Seddon KR, Rehmann L. Disruption and wet extraction of the microalgae Chlorella vulgaris using room-temperature ionic liquids. ACS Sustainable Chemistry & Engineering. 2016;**4**:591-600

[84] Kong M, Wang F, Tian L, Tang H, Zhang L. Functional identification of glutamate cysteine ligase and glutathione synthetase in the marine yeast Rhodosporidium diobovatum. Naturwissenschaften. 2017;**105**(1-2):4

[85] Pompella A, Visvikis A, Paolicchi A, De Tata V, Casini AF. The changing faces of glutathione, a cellular protagonist. Biochemical Pharmacology. 2003;**66**(8):1499-1503

[86] Civiero E, Pintus M, Ruggeri C, Tamburini E, Sollai F, Sanjust E, et al. Physiological and phylogenetic characterization of Rhodotorula diobovata DSBCA06, a Nitrophilous yeast. Biology (Basel). 2018;**7**(3):39

[87] Jiru TM, Steyn L, Pohl C, Abate D. Production of single cell oil from cane molasses by Rhodotorula kratochvilovae (syn, Rhodosporidium kratochvilovae) SY89 as a biodiesel feedstock. Chemistry Central Journal. 2018;**12**(1):91

[88] Jiru TM, Abate D, Kiggundu N, Pohl C, Groenewald M. Oleaginous yeasts from Ethiopia. AMB Express. 2016;**6**(1):78

[89] Jiru TM, Groenewald M, Pohl C, Steyn L, Kiggundu N, Abate D. Optimization of cultivation conditions for biotechnological production of lipid by Rhodotorula kratochvilovae (syn, Rhodosporidium kratochvilovae) SY89 for biodiesel preparation. 3 Biotech. 2017;**7**(2):145

[90] Galafassi S, Cucchetti D, Pizza F, Franzosi G, Bianchi D, Compagno C. Lipid production for second generation biodiesel by the oleaginous yeast Rhodotorula graminis. Bioresource Technology. 2012;**111**:398-403

[91] Breierova E, Certik M, Marova I, Vadkertiova R. The effect of Zn(II) ions and reactive oxygen on the uptake of zinc and production of carotenoids by selected red yeasts. Chemistry & Biodiversity. 2018;**15**(6):e1800069

[92] Du C, Li Y, Guo Y, Han M, Zhang W, Qian H. The suppression of torulene and torularhodin treatment on the growth of PC-3 xenograft prostate tumors. Biochemical and Biophysical Research Communications. 2016;**469**(4):1146-1152

[93] Ungureanu C, Ferdes M. Evaluation of antioxidant and antimicrobial activities of Torularhodin. Advanced Science Letters. 2012;**18**:50-53

[94] Kot AM, Blazejak S, Gientka I, Kieliszek M, Brys J. Torulene and torularhodin: "new" fungal carotenoids for industry? Microbial Cell Factories. 2018;**17**(1):49

[95] Miccoli C, Palmieri D, De Curtis F, Lima G, Ianiri G, Castoria R. Complete genome sequence of the biocontrol agent yeast Rhodotorula kratochvilovae strain LS11. Genome Announcements. 2018;**6**(10):e00120-e00118

[96] De Curtis F. I Lieviti Nella Lotta Biologica Contro Patogeni Fungini Degli Ortofrutticoli in Postraccolta: Attività e Meccanismi D'azione Coinvolti. Bologna, Italy: University of Bologna; 1998

[97] Pinedo C, Wright SAI, Collado IG, Goss RJM, Castoria R, Hrelia P, et al. Isotopic labeling studies reveal the Patulin detoxification pathway by the biocontrol yeast Rhodotorula kratochvilovae LS11. Journal of Natural Products. 2018;**81**:2692-2699

[98] Buck JW. Combinations of fungicides with Phylloplane yeasts for improved control of Botrytis cinerea on Geranium seedlings. Phytopathology. 2004;**94**(2):196-202

[99] Orndorff SA, Costantino N, Stewart D, Durham DR. Strain improvement of Rhodotorula graminis for production of a novel l-phenylalanine Ammonia-Lyase. Applied and Environmental Microbiology. 1988;**54**(4):996-1002

[100] Rowles I, Groenendaal B, Binay B, Malone KJ, Willies SC, Turner NJ. Engineering of phenylalanine ammonia lyase from Rhodotorula graminis for the enhanced synthesis of unnatural L-amino acids. Tetrahedron. 2016;**72**:7343-7347

[101] Cajka T, Garay LA, Sitepu IR, Boundy-Mills KL, Fiehn O. Multiplatform mass spectrometry-based approach identifies extracellular glycolipids of the yeast *Rhodotorula babjevae* UCDFST 04-877. Journal of Natural Products. 2016;**79**(10):2580-2589

[102] Garay LA, Sitepu IR, Cajka T, Fiehn O, Cathcart E, Fry RW, et al. Discovery of synthesis and secretion of polyol esters of fatty acids by four basidiomycetous yeast species in the order Sporidiobolales. Journal of Industrial Microbiology & Biotechnology. 2017;**44**:923-936

[103] Tulloch A, Spencer J. Extracellular glycolipids of Rhodotorula species. Canadian Journal of Chemistry. 1964;**42**:830-835

[104] Pasquali RC, Taurozzi MP, Bregni C. Some considerations about the hydrophilic-lipophilic balance system. International Journal of Pharmaceutics. 2008;**356**(1-2):44-51

[105] Griffin W. Classification of surface-active agents by HLB. Journal of the Society of Cosmetic Chemists. 1949;**1**(5):311-326

[106] Yamashita Y, Sakamoto K. Hydrophilic–lipophilic balance (HLB): Classical indexation and novel indexation of surfactant. In: Encyclopedia of Biocolloid and Biointerface Science. Hoboken, NJ, USA: John Wiley & Sons Inc; 2016

[107] Davies J. London. 1957. http://citeseerx.ist.psu.edu/viewdoc/download?doi=10.1.1.473.424&rep=rep1&type=pdf

[108] Lyman M, Rubinfeld B, Leif R, Mulcahy H, Dugan L, Souza B. *Rhodotorula taiwanensis* MD1149 produces hypoacetylated PEFA compounds with increased surface activity compared to *Rhodotorula babjevae* MD1169. PLoS One. 2018;**13**(1):e0190373

[109] Tkavc R, Matrosova VY, Grichenko OE, Gostincar C, Volpe RP, Klimenkova P, et al. Prospects for fungal bioremediation of acidic radioactive waste sites: Characterization and genome sequence of *Rhodotorula taiwanensis* MD1149. Frontiers in Microbiology. 2017;**8**:2528

Chapter 7

De Novo Synthesis of Plant Natural Products in Yeast

Wentao Sun, Yu-jia Zhao and Chun Li

Abstract

Plant natural products possess versatile biological activities including antiviral, anticancer and hepatoprotective activities, which are widely used in pharmaceutical and many other health-related fields. However, current production of such compounds relies on plant culture and extraction, which brings about severe concerns for environmental, ecological and amount of agricultural lands used. With the increasing awareness of environmental sustainability and shortage of lands, yeasts are engineered to produce natural products, for its inherent advantages such as the robustness, safety and sufficient supply of precursors. This chapter focused on the recent progress of yeast as a platform for the biosynthesis of plant natural products.

Keywords: natural products, flavonoids, alkaloids, terpenoids, terpenoids saponins, biomanufacturing, heterogeneous synthesis, yeast

1. Introduction

Plant natural products were a kind of active compounds including flavonoids, alkaloids, terpenoids and saponins etc. As the main composition of plants secondary metabolites, these compounds play an important role in plant communication and defensing, so these compounds have been widely used as herbicide and pesticide in the agricultural industry [1]. For example, oleanane saponins isolated from *Bellis sylvestris* exhibit strong phytotoxic activity against Aegilops geniculate, and saponins from alfalfa can cause a decrease of food metabolized by *Tenebrio molitor* [2]. These compounds were also the major bioactive constituents of some traditional herbal medicines, such as ginsenosides from ginseng and glycyrrhizin from licorice. In addition, some natural products possess special flavors. For instance, camphor alcohol has distinctive aroma, while glycyrrhetinic acid monoglucuronide and mogroside V have a strong sweetness which are approximately 941-fold and 300-fold of sucrose, respectively [3]. These sweet tasting compounds have been widely used in the food industries for weight loss. As a kind of amphiphilic compounds, saponins can also act as robust foaming agent in aqueous solutions. Based on this trait potential, they have been explored in the cosmetics and detergent industries.

Currently, the production of natural products are mainly based on extraction from plants, which is a low yield, time consuming, labor intensive and environment unfriendly supply way [4]. The inefficient approach could not match the huge demands of market, and further limit the application of these compounds in the pharmaceutical, agricultural, food, cosmetic and detergent industries. Thus, developing novel approaches are of great significance to replace the traditional method.

Producing natural products via microorganism cell factories turned out to be a promising solution. Compared with plants, microbes exhibit many advantages, including fast growing, land saving and controllable. Yeast especially *Saccharomyces cerevisiae* (*S. cerevisiae*) has become a widely used host for producing these products because of its similar intracellular structure with plant cells, such as the inherent endomembrane system for microsomal enzymes to stand on. Moreover, the generally recognized as safe (GRAS) yeast as a robust industrial strain is widely used in food and alcohol production and has a clear genetic background. Typically, nearly 25 g/L artemisinic acid has been produced in *S. cerevisiae*, which indicated that producing natural products by yeast is a potential approach to substitute the traditional supply way.

In this chapter, we systematically illustrate the decoded biosynthetic pathway of flavonoids, alkaloids, terpenoids and terpenoids saponins assisted by yeast. Then briefly summarize the progress of yeast to produce plant natural products. Furthermore, novel strategies and tools used to boost their production were discussed.

2. Synthetic pathways of natural products

Flavonoids and alkaloids are usually derived from the shikimate pathway, which exists in prokaryotic, eukaryotic, and archaeal microorganisms. The synthesis pathway start from the stereo-specific condensation catalyzed by 3-deoxy-Darabino-heptulosonate-7-phosphate synthase to generate 3-deoxy-Darabino-heptulosonate-7-phosphate (DAHP), which is further catalyzed to form chorismate a common precursor for various aromatic compounds, including aromatic amino acids, then these aromatic compound will be converted to flavonoids and alkaloids **Figure 1(a)**.

Terpenes and saponins are usually synthesized from the common five-carbon building blocks, 3-isopentenyl pyrophosphate (IPP) and dimethylallyl pyrophosphate (DMAPP), which are synthesized through mevalonic acid (MVA) or 2-C-methyl-D-erythritol 4-phosphate (MEP) pathway [5]. These five-carbon units are condensed to geranyl pyrophosphate (GPP), geranylgeranyl pyrophosphate (GGPP), and farnesyl pyrophosphate (FPP). These precursors are then diverted to specialized terpenes by terpene synthases. GPP is converted to monoterpene by

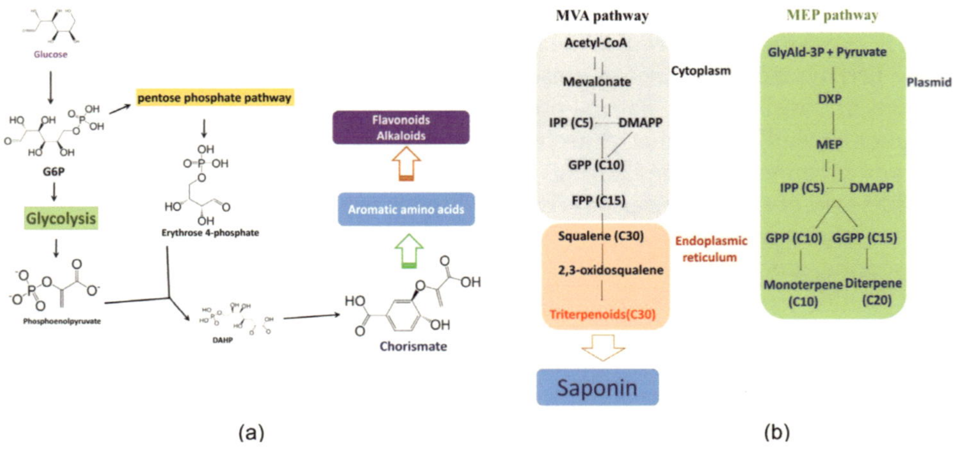

Figure 1.
(a) Scheme for flavonoid and alkaloid biosynthetic pathways. (b) Scheme for terpene and saponins biosynthetic pathways.

monoterpene synthases, GGPP were used to synthesize diterpenes which can be further converted to tretaterpenes, and FPP is the precursor for triterpenes which can be converted to saponins by UGTs **Figure 1(b)**.

In order to produce flavonoids, alkaloids, monoterpene, diterpene and tretaterpene heterogeneously, *E. coli* is widely used for enzyme identification, because of its ease genetic manipulations, whereas the yeast platform was mostly used in triterpene synthesis for its endogenous 2,3-oxidosqualene supplement and inner membrane structure for membrane located plant CYP450 to stand on, which is intensively used and studied in natural products synthesis.

During triterpenoids synthesis, FPP is condensed to 2,3-oxidosqualene, which is subsequently cyclized to polycyclic triterpenoid skeletons by oxidosqualene cyclases (OSCs). These molecules are oxidized by CYP450s forming aglycones, which are further glycosylated to triterpenoid saponins by UGTs.

Cyclization of 2,3-oxidosqualene by OSCs, was the first step in triterpenoid biosynthesis. Because of the efficient 2,3-oxidosqualene supplement, most OSCs was verified by directly expressing in yeast [6]. Plants OSCs always possess promiscuous activities, and could cyclize 2,3-oxidosqualene to different conformations simultaneously. For example, amyrin synthase from *Glycyrrhiza uralensis* can produce not only α-amyrin but also β-amyrin [7]. Due to the multiple-activity of OSCs, more than 100 kinds of triterpenoid skeletons could be generated during cyclization. This was considered as a part of plant defense, for many defensive substances could be produced by one process, which can alleviate the metabolic burden of the plants. However, the promiscuity of OSCs would lead to undesired structural analogue [8].

The triterpenoid skeletons could be further oxidized by CYP450s, introducing active groups such as hydroxyl, carboxyl or epoxy groups [9]. The CYP450s decoding process was complicated, for the identification of CYP450s need much chemical and bioinformatics information, and the membrane located plant CYP450s is hard to express in *E. coli*. Hence, *S. cerevisiae* together with chromatography mass spectrum and NMR play an important role in the decoding of plant biosynthetic pathways involving CYP450s especially for the biosynthesis of triterpenoids and their saponins. To date, 48 CYP450s have been identified involved in triterpenoid saponins biosynthesis. They were summarized in **Table 1**.

No.	Name	Accession number	Plant species	Substrate	Loci
1	CYP51H10	ABG88965.1	*Avena strigosa*	β-amyrin	C-12, 13, 16β
2	CYP71D353	AHB62239.1	*Lotus japonicus*	lupeol	C-20
3	CYP72A61v2	BAL45199.1	*Medicago truncatula*	24-OH-β-amyrin	C-23
4	CYP72A63	BAL45200.1	*Medicago truncatula*	β-amyrin	C-30
5	CYP72A67	ABC59075.1	*Medicago truncatula*	oleanolic acid	C-2
6	CYP72A68v2	BAL45204.1	*Medicago truncatula*	oleanolic acid	C-25
7	CYP72A69	BAW35014.1	*Glycine max*	β-amyrin	C-21
8	CYP72A154	BAL45207.1	*Glycyrrhiza uralensis*	β-amyrin	C-30
9	CYP87D16	AHF22090.1	*Maesa lanceolata*	β-amyrin	C-16α
10	CYP88D6	AQQ13664.1	*Glycyrrhiza uralensis*	β-amyrin	C-11
11	CYP93E1	BAE94181.1	*Glycine max*	β-amyrin	C-24
12	CYP93E2	ABC59085.1	*Medicago truncatula*	β-amyrin	C-24

No.	Name	Accession number	Plant species	Substrate	Loci
13	CYP93E3	BAG68930.1	*Glycyrrhiza uralensis*	β-amyrin	C-24
14	CYP93E4	AIN25416.1	*Arachis hypogaea*	β-amyrin	C-24
15	CYP93E5	AIN25417.1	*Cicer arietinum*	β-amyrin	C-24
16	CYP93E6	AIN25418.1	*Glycyrrhiza glabra*	β-amyrin	C-24
17	CYP93E7	AIN25419.1	*Lens culinaris*	β-amyrin	C-24
18	CYP93E8	AIN25420.1	*Pisum sativum*	β-amyrin	C-24
19	CYP93E9	AIN25421.1	*Phaseolus vulgaris*	β-amyrin	C-24
20	CYP716A12	ABC59076.1	*Medicago truncatula*	α-amyrin, β-amyrin, lupeol	C-28
21	CYP716A14v2	AHF22083.1	*Artemisia annua*	α-amyrin, β-amyrin	C-3
22	CYP716A15	BAJ84106.1	*Vitis vinifera*	α-amyrin, β-amyrin, lupeol	C-28
23	CYP716A17	BAJ84107.1	*Vitis vinifera*	α-amyrin, β-amyrin, lupeol	C-28
24	CYP716A44	–	*Solanum lycopersicum*	α-amyrin, β-amyrin	C-28
25	CYP716A46	–	*Solanum lycopersicum*	α-amyrin, β-amyrin	C-28
26	CYP716A47	AEY75213.1	*Panax ginseng*	dammarenediol-II	C-12
27	CYP716A52v2	AFO63032.1	*Panax ginseng*	β-amyrin	C-28
28	CYP716A53v2	AFO63031.1	*Panax ginseng*	dammarenediol-II	C-20
29	CYP716A75	AHF22088.1	*Maesa lanceolata*	β-amyrin	C-28
30	CYP716A78	ANY30853.1	*Chenopodium quinoa*	α-amyrin, β-amyrin, lupeol	C-28
31	CYP716A79	ANY30854.1	*Chenopodium quinoa*	α-amyrin, β-amyrin, lupeol	C-28
32	CYP716A80	ALR73782.1	*Barbarea vulgaris*	α-amyrin, β-amyrin, lupeol	C-28
33	CYP716A81	ALR73781.1	*Barbarea vulgaris*	α-amyrin, β-amyrin, lupeol	C-28
34	CYP716A83	AOG74832.1	*Centella asiatica*	β-amyrin	C-28
35	CYP716A86	AOG74831.1	*Centella asiatica*	β-amyrin	C-28
36	CYP716A140	AOG74836.1	*Platycodon grandiflorus*	β-amyrin, 24-OH-β-amyrin	C-28
37	CYP716A141	AOG74838.1	*Platycodon grandiflorus*	β-amyrin, 24-OH-β-amyrin	C-28
38	CYP716A180	–	*Betula platyphylla*	lupeol	C-28
39	CYP716A244	APZ88353.1	*Eleutherococcus senticosus*	β-amyrin	C-28
40	CYP716A254	–	*Anemone flaccida*	β-amyrin	C-28
41	CYP716AL1	AEX07773.1	*Catharanthus roseus*	α-amyrin, β-amyrin, lupeol	C-28
42	CYP716C11	AOG74835.1	*Centella asiatica*	oleanolic acid	C-2
43	CYP716E41	AOG74834.1	*Centella asiatica*	maslinic acid	C-6

No.	Name	Accession number	Plant species	Substrate	Loci
44	CYP716E22	–	*Solanum lycopersicum*	α-amyrin, β-amyrin	C-6
45	CYP716S5	AOG74839.1	*Platycodon grandiflorus*	β-amyrin, oleanolic acid	C-12, 13
46	CYP716Y1	AHF45909.1	*Bupleurum falcatum*	α-amyrin, β-amyrin	C-16α
47	CYP716A1	AED94045.1	*Arabidopsis thaliana*	β-amyrin	C-28
48	CYP716A2	BAU61505.1	*Arabidopsis thaliana*	α-amyrin	C-22

Table 1.
Overview of plant CYP450s in triterpenoid saponins biosynthesis.

Glycosylation is the last step of triterpenoid saponins biosynthesis that links hydrophilic sugar moieties to the hydrophobic aglycone by UGTs. By glycosylation, various monosaccharide units (including glucose, glucuronic acid, galactose, rhamnose, xylose and arabinose, etc.) could be linked to aglycone at the positions C-3, C-28, C-4, C-16, C-20, C-21, C-22 and/or C-23. The introduced of sugar moieties could improve triterpenoid saponins bioactivities. In view of the tremendous amounts of UGTs in plants, more than 120 genes encoding family 1 UGTs have been identified in *Arabidopsis thaliana* genome [10]. However, Decoding the specific UGT involved in target triterpenoid saponins biosynthesis was very difficult. So far, only 23 UGTs have been identified, which involved in triterpenoid saponins biosynthesis. They were summarized in **Table 2**.

No.	Name	Accession number	Plant species	Substrate	Loci
1	UGT71G1	AAW56092.1	*Medicago truncatula*	Medicagenic acid UDP- glucose	C-3, 28
2	UGT73AD1	ALD84259.1	*Centella asiatica*	Asiatic acid, Madecassic acid UDP- glucose	C-28
3	UGT73AE1	AJT58578.1	*Carthamus tinctorius*	Glycyrrhetinic acid UDP- glucose	C-3
4	UGT73AH1	AUR26623.1	*Centella asiatica*	Asiatic Acid UDP- glucose	C-28
5	UGT73C10	AFN26666.1	*Barbarea vulgaris*	Hederagenin, Oleanolic acid UDP- glucose	C-3
6	UGT73C11	AFN26667.1	*Barbarea vulgaris*	Glycyrrhetinic acid, Oleanolic acid UDP- glucose	C-3
7	UGT73C12	AFN26668.1	*Barbarea vulgaris*	Hederagenin, Oleanolic acid UDP- glucose	C-3
8	UGT73C13	AFN26669.1	*Barbarea vulgaris*	Hederagenin, Oleanolic acid UDP-glucose	C-3
9	UGT73F2	BAM29362.1	*Glycine max*	Saponin A0-gα UDP-xylose	C-22
10	UGT73F3	ACT34898.1	*Medicago truncatula*	Hederagenin UDP- glucose	C-28
11	UGT73F4	BAM29363.1	*Glycine max*	Saponin A0-gα UDP-xylose	C-22
12	UGT73F17	AXS75258.	*Glycyrrhiza uralensis*	Glycyrrhizin UDP-glucose	C-30

No.	Name	Accession number	Plant species	Substrate	Loci
13	UGT73K1	AAW56091.1	*Medicago truncatula*	Hederagenin, Soyasapogenols B and E UDP-glucose	C-3, 28
14	UGT74AE2	–	*Panax Quinquefolium*	Protopanaxadiol UDP-glucose	C-3
15	UGT74M1	ABK76266.1	*Vaccaria hispanica*	Gypsogenic acid UDP-glucose	C-28
16	UGT94Q2	–	*Panax Quinquefolium*	Ginsenoside Rh2 UDP-glucose	C-3
17	UGTPg1	–	*Panax ginseng*	Protopanaxadiol UDP-glucose	C-3
18	UGTPg100	–	*Panax ginseng*	Ginsenoside RF1, Protopanaxatriol UDP-glucose	C-6
19	UGTPg101	–	*Panax ginseng*	Ginsenoside RF1, Protopanaxatriol UDP-glucose	C-6, 20
20	Pg3-O-UGT1	–	*Panax quinquefolius*	Protopanaxadiol UDP-glucose	C-3
21	GmSGT2	BAI99584.1	*Glycine max*	Soyasapogenol B monoglucuronide UDP-galactose	C-3
22	GmSGT3	BAI99585.1	*Glycine max*	Soyasaponin III UDP-rhamnose	C-3
23	UDPG	–	*Panax ginseng*	Ginsenoside Rd. UDP-glucose	

Table 2.
Overview of plant UGTs in triterpenoid saponins biosynthesis.

3. Biosynthesis of natural products in yeast

3.1 Biosynthesis of flavonoids in yeast

Flavonoids are among the most extensively investigated natural products, which could be divided into several subgroups, including common flavonoids (e.g., galangin, eriodictyol, catechin, quercetin, luteolin, myricetin and cyanidin), isoflavonoids (e.g., genistein) and neoflavonoids (e.g., calophyllolide, isodispar B). Due to their physiological activity and decoded synthesis pathways, the heterologous biosynthesis of flavonoids and their derivatives, have been extensively studied in microbial hosts mostly in *E. coli*. However, high-level flavonoids could also be produced by yeast [11].

Based on yeast platform, 531 mg/L resveratrol production was achieved via the tyrosine pathway directly using glucose and ethanol as substrate in fed-batch fermentation. Through the subsequent pull-push-block strain engineering strategy, more resveratrol production formed via the phenylalanine pathway increased up to 800 mg/L directly from glucose which was the highest titer of resveratrol up to now.

The co-culture system was also developed for flavonoids production. In the collaboration system of *E. coli* and yeast to produce naringenin, *E. coli* provides precursors tyrosine and acetate for yeast to produce naringenin, and finally 21.16 mg/L naringenin was obtained from xylose.

3.2 Biosynthesis of alkaloids in yeast

Alkaloid compounds, especially plant-derived benzylisoquinoline alkaloids and monoterpene indole alkaloids are considered as a valuable source of pharmaceuticals for its anticancer, antiviral and antimalarial activities, et al. In order to replace plant-extracting method, the reconstruction of plant-derived alkaloid biosynthetic pathways in microbes are extensively studied. Though always achieve much lower titers than in *E. coli*, yeast platform was used to produce alkaloid with complex pathway.

By overexpressing 14 known monoterpene indole alkaloid pathway genes and an enhancement of secondary metabolism through overexpression of additional seven genes and deletion of three genes, strictosidine was produced in yeast with a production of 0.53 mg/L. (S)-reticuline (around 80 μg/L), baine (6.4 μg/L) and hydrocodone (0.3 μg/L) have been produced in yeast from simple sugars. Indeed, the titers was low; However, very recently, the total assembly and optimization of the noscapine biosynthetic pathway involving over 30 enzymes in yeast was realized, which was very hard to reconstruct in *E. coli*, and led to a final titer of 2.2 mg/L noscapine using sugars as substrate [12].

3.3 Biosynthesis of terpenes and saponins in yeast

Similar with flavonoids and alkaloids, some simple terpenoids skeletons such as monoterpenoid and diterpenoid, which were produced directly by terpenoid synthase, were mostly studied in *E. coli* for the high activity and easy expression of these terpenoid synthase in *E. coli*. However, in recent years, yeast hosts also attracted more and more attention in these fields.

By expressing geraniol synthase from *Ocimum basilicum*, 0.5 mg/L geraniol was obtained in the engineered yeast. The inefficient supplement of precursors GPP should be responsible for the low production. To improve the final geraniol concentration, an ERG20 mutant was used to block the competitive pathway and the production was improved to 5 mg/L. Based on the inherent GPP and the blocking of the competitive FPP synthesis pathway, other volatile monoterpenes, including sabinene and limonene, were also produced by expressing plant monoterpene synthase in yeast host.

Moreover, the heterologous biosynthesis of diterpenoid by yeast also became a new trend and gained more and more attention. Through introducing diterpenoids synthase and metabolic optimization, several plant diterpenoids including taxadiene and miltiradiene were produced in yeast. With the introducing of the taxadiene biosynthetic pathways, and the optimization of precursors supplement by strengthen the MVA pathway through overexpressing tHMG1 and UPC2-1 (a global transcription factor of MVA), the taxadiene was successfully produce in the engineered yeast and achieved a production of 8.7 mg/L, though the production was lower than that produced in *E. coli* (1 g/L). However, when it involves in more complex skeletons, such as ferruginol and carnosic acid which need further oxidation by CYP450s, yeast displays the huge potential. The membrane located plant CYP450s are hard to functionally expressed in *E. coli*. By co-expressing CYP76AH1 and plant cytochrome P450 reductase (CPR) genes heterogeneously in a miltiradiene producing yeast strain, ferruginol was successfully achieved with a titer of 10.5 mg/L. Based on ferruginol, carnosic acid, a C20 oxidations products of miltiradiene, was produced in yeast by introducing an extra CYP76AK6-8 and these compounds still cannot be produced by *E. coli*.

As an exception, the heterogeneous biosynthesis of triterpenoid and triterpenoid saponins were mostly studied in yeast, for the membrane located plant OSC and CYP450 are challengeable to correctly express in *E. coli*. By overexpressing the codon optimized OSC from *Glycyrrhiza glabra* designated as β-amyrin synthase (βAS), Zhang et al. obtained a β-amyrin production as high as 138.8 mg/L in the engineered *S. cerevisiae* Sgib [13]. Through co-expressing the liquorice CYP88D6 and CYP72A154 with β-amyrin synthase and CPR genes in yeast, glycyrrhetinic acid was produced with a titer of about 20 μg/L. To boost the glycyrrhetinic acid titer, Zhu et al identified novel CYP450s uni25647 and CYP72A63 with higher activity than CYP88D6 and CYP72A154 by yeast host. With these two CYP450s and a novel liquorice CPR, Zhu et al. reconstructed the GA synthesis pathway in sgib and improved the glycyrrhetinic acid titer up to 18.9 mg/L, which is 1000 folds compared with that in the former study [14]. Zhao et al. overexpressed an efficient CPR (MtCPR1) gene, and reconstructed the galactose regulatory network by knocking out GAL1 and GAL80 while using strong inducible promoters GAL1 and GAL10 to operate CYPP450, MtCPR1, ERG1 and ERG9). Finally, 186.1 mg/L oleanic acid was achieved in yeast, which is the highest concentration in reported literatures [15]. More recently, Yu et al. introduced a high specific α-amyrin synthase in yeast leading to the production of α-amyrin, β-amyrin and lupeol at a ratio of 86:13:1 with the α-amyrin titer of 11.97 mg/L, 5.8-folds of the maximum production reported [16].

Benefit from the yeast hosts, the more complex saponins were also heterologously synthesized. By expressing *Barbarea vulgaris* UGT73C11 in a glycyrrhetinic acid producing yeast strain, Liu et al. realized the de novo synthesis of glycyrrhetinic acid-3-O-monoglucose starting from sample glucose [17]. With the decoding of plant biosynthetic pathways, many other triterpenoid saponins have been successfully synthesized in yeast factories and the high production of ginsenoside Rh2 (2.5 g/L) has highlighted the commercial feasibility of this approach.

Panax ginseng is a famous herb medicine widely used in Asia, which possesses various pharmaceutical activities including anticancer, anti-inflammatory and antiviral activities. These activities are mainly endowed by its triterpenoids saponins, known as ginsenosides [18]. Because of their low content and the long culture cycle of ginseng, the heterologous biosynthesis of ginsenosides in microbial cell factories is drawing more and more attention. To date, various ginsenosides and its aglycones have been successfully produced in *S. cerevisiae* (**Figure 2**), including protopanaxadiol, protopanaxatriol and oleanolic acid, the three main kinds of aglycones, and four kinds of ginsenosides, ginsenosides Rh2, Rg3, RF1 and Rh1. In addition, some unnatural ginsenosides such as compound K and 3β, 12β-Di-O-Glc-PPD have also been synthesized by combination various enzymes from different species.

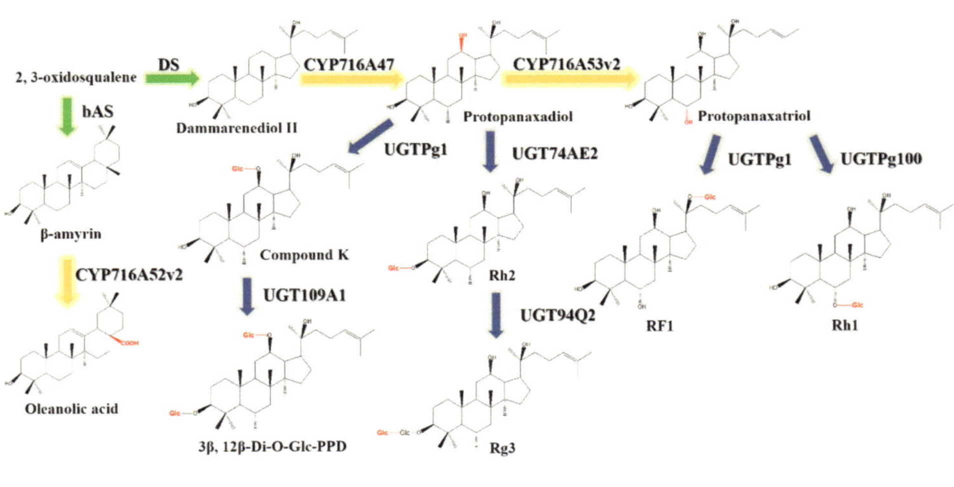

Figure 2.
Scheme for ginsenosides biosynthesized in S. cerevisiae. The green arrows represent OSCs, the yellow arrows represent CYP450s, the blue arrows represent UGTs.

Protopanaxadiol (PPD) is an important starting material for the biosynthesis of ginsenoside, which is synthesized from 2,3-oxidosqualene by dammarenediol-II synthase and CYP450s. Through expressing *P. ginseng* dammarenediol-II synthase (PgDS), *P. ginseng* CYP716A47 and *A. thaliana* CYP450 reductase 1 (AtCPR1), PPD was firstly produced in *S. cerevisiae* [19]. Subsequently, the more complex ginsenosides aglycone protopanaxatriol (PPT) was produced by engineered yeast carrying *P. ginseng* CYP716A53v2 and AtCPR1 which uses PPD as substrate. By the similar strategy of co-expression of *P. ginseng* β-amyrin synthase (PNY1) CYP716A52v2 and AtCPR1, oleanolic acid (OA), a oleanane-type pentacyclic triterpene, was synthesized in *S. cerevisiae* [20]. Although these three ginsenoside aglycones had been successfully synthesized in yeast, the titer was still too low. A truncated version of tHMG1 (3-hydroxyl-3-methylglutaryl-CoA reductase), ERG20 (farnesyl diphosphate synthase), ERG9 (squalene synthase) and ERG1 (2,3-oxidosqualene synthase) were overexpressed to improve the PPD production in *S. cerevisiae*. Together with a codon optimized *P. ginseng* CYP716A53v2, the production of PPD was increased by 262-fold and up to nearly 1.2 g/L. The efficient supplement of PPD made the strain an ideal platform for further tailored ginsenosides biosynthesis [21]. By similar strategies, the PPT production was increased by overexpressing *ERG9*, *ERG1*, *tHMG1* and corresponding CYP450 genes with codon optimization.

The widely studied ginsenosides Rh2 and Rg3 which are synthesized from PPD have been successfully biosynthesized in *S. cerevisiae*. By expressing PgDS, CYP450 system consisting of CYP716A47, AtCPR2 to supply PPD, and the co-expressing of PgUGT74AE2 and PgUGT94Q2 for glycosylation of PPD, Rg3 was heterologously synthesized in *S. cerevisiae*. Combine with the approach of replacing the native promoter of ERG7 with a methionine-repressible promoter (MET3), the production of Rg3 was increased up to 1.3 mg/L. [22] Other type of ginsenosides such as RF1 and Rh1 were synthesized through the co-expression of PgDS, CYP716A53v2, CYP716A47, PgCPR1 and UGTPg100 (or UGTPg1). The production of RF1 and Rh1 reached 42.1 and 92.8 mg/L in *S. cerevisiae*, respectively [23].

It is demonstrated that compound K (CK), generally considered as the metabolite of glycosidases [24], is the main functional form of oral administration of ginsenosides [25]. By the co-expression of PgDS, AtCPR2, CYP716A47 and UGTPg1, CK has already been synthesized in *S. cerevisiae*. Its production was further increased up to 1.4 mg/L by overexpressing tHMG1 and UPC2.1 as well as controlling heterogeneous genes via GAL promoters [26]. By combination of tailoring enzymes from various species, more unnatural ginsenosides could be synthesized in *S. cerevisiae*. Through the combination of plant PgDS, CYP716A47, AtCPR1 and UGT109A1 from *B. subtilis*, 3β, 12β-Di-O-Glc-PPD was produced in *S. cerevisiae*. To further optimize the production, overexpression of tHMG1 and the fusion expression PgDS was carried out, and ERG7 (encoding lanosterol synthase) promoter was replaced with an antisense one. Through these strategies, the production of 3β,12β-Di-O-Glc-PPD was increased up to 9.05 mg/L in the engineered *S. cerevisiae* [27].

Besides ginsenosides, the heterogeneous biosynthesis of other triterpenoids saponins with markedly physiological function also attracted much attention. The natural sweeter mogroside V from S. grosvenorii, which is nearly 300 times sweeter than sucrose, is widely used as a food additive in low-calorie sweet beverages [28]. Through analysis of S. grosvenorii transcriptome data and gene mining, the key genes involved in mogroside V synthesis including cycloartenol synthase (CAS) gene, epoxide hydrolases (EPH) gene, CYP102801, UGT94-289-3 and UGT720-269-1 have been identified. By introducing these enzymes together with squalene synthase (SQS), squalene epoxidase (SQE) and AtCPR1 in *S. cerevisiae*, mogroside V was successfully produced. These advances highlight the possibility to produce natural, noncaloric sweetener mogrosides by engineered yeast.

Saikosaponins are the major pharmaceutical constituents of *B. falcatum*, an important perennial herb widely used in traditional Chinese medicine which exert multiple bioactivities [29]. Currently, two saikosaponins aglycones, 16α-hydroxy α-amyrin and 16α-hydroxy β-amyrin have been synthesized in engineered *S. cerevisiae* through co-expressing CYP716Y1, AtCTR1, CaDDS (dammarenediol synthase from *Centella asiatica*) or GgbAS (β-amyrin synthase from *Glycyrrhiza glabra* in *S. cerevisiae*, respectively [30].

Moreover, by overexpressing lycopene synthetic genes from *Erwinia uredovora*, this ungroomed tetraterpene compound was synthesized by the engineered yeast strain, with a production of 3.3 mg/g CDW. To boost the lycopene production in yeast, Ma et al. overexpressed key genes associated with fatty acid synthesis, TAG production, and TAG fatty acyl composition, and deleted FLD1 to increase lipid-droplet size for more hydrophobic storage space of lycopene, leading to a production of 2.37 g/L, which weighed against that produced in *E. coli* [31]. This indicates the potential of yeast to produce simple terpenoid directly synthesized by terpenoid synthase.

All these progresses indicate the great potential of yeast for heterologous synthesis of natural products, especially for these with complex molecular structure and synthetic pathways such as terpenoids and their saponins. Recently, various kinds of terpenoids and saponins were heterologously produced in yeast, but most of them had a low final concentration far from to instead of plant extracting methods. To boost the production efficiency of engineered yeast strains, various strategies need intensively study.

4. Strategies for boosting biosynthesis of terpenoids in yeast

Although various kinds of natural products could be produced by yeast, many challenges still remain for this approach. The main bottleneck of building an efficient yeast cell factory was that the biosynthetic pathways are not totally elucidated and the poor or disappeared activity of plant enzymes when expressed in yeast. Moreover, the destabilization on the native metabolic flux caused by the heterogeneous pathways could lead to low cell growth and low final products concentration, and the cytotoxicity most of natural products also restrict the use of microbial hosts for producing natural products. Strategies and biotools focused on settling such issues to accelerate the microbial natural products biosynthesis in yeast host have been developed based on omics, metabolic engineering and protein engineering (**Figure 3**).

4.1 Strategies to redesign natural biosynthetic pathways

Unlike some prokaryotic biosynthetic pathway genes, which always locate on a gene cluster, the genes involved in triterpenoid saponins biosynthesis always distributes among the whole genome in plants. Moreover, the expression of these genes generally needs intricate inducible conditions, which increase the difficulty to elucidate triterpenoid saponins biosynthetic pathways.

Benefit from the rapid progress of sequencing technology, genome and transcriptome of many medicinal plants have been sequenced, and the information has been publicly available online (http://medicinalplantgenomics.msu.edu). The analysis of the genome and transcriptome date facilitates the prediction of genes involved in the targeted compound biosynthesis. Through the comparison of the transcriptome information between plants or tissues with high- and low-production of the target compounds, several key genes could be predicted. For example,

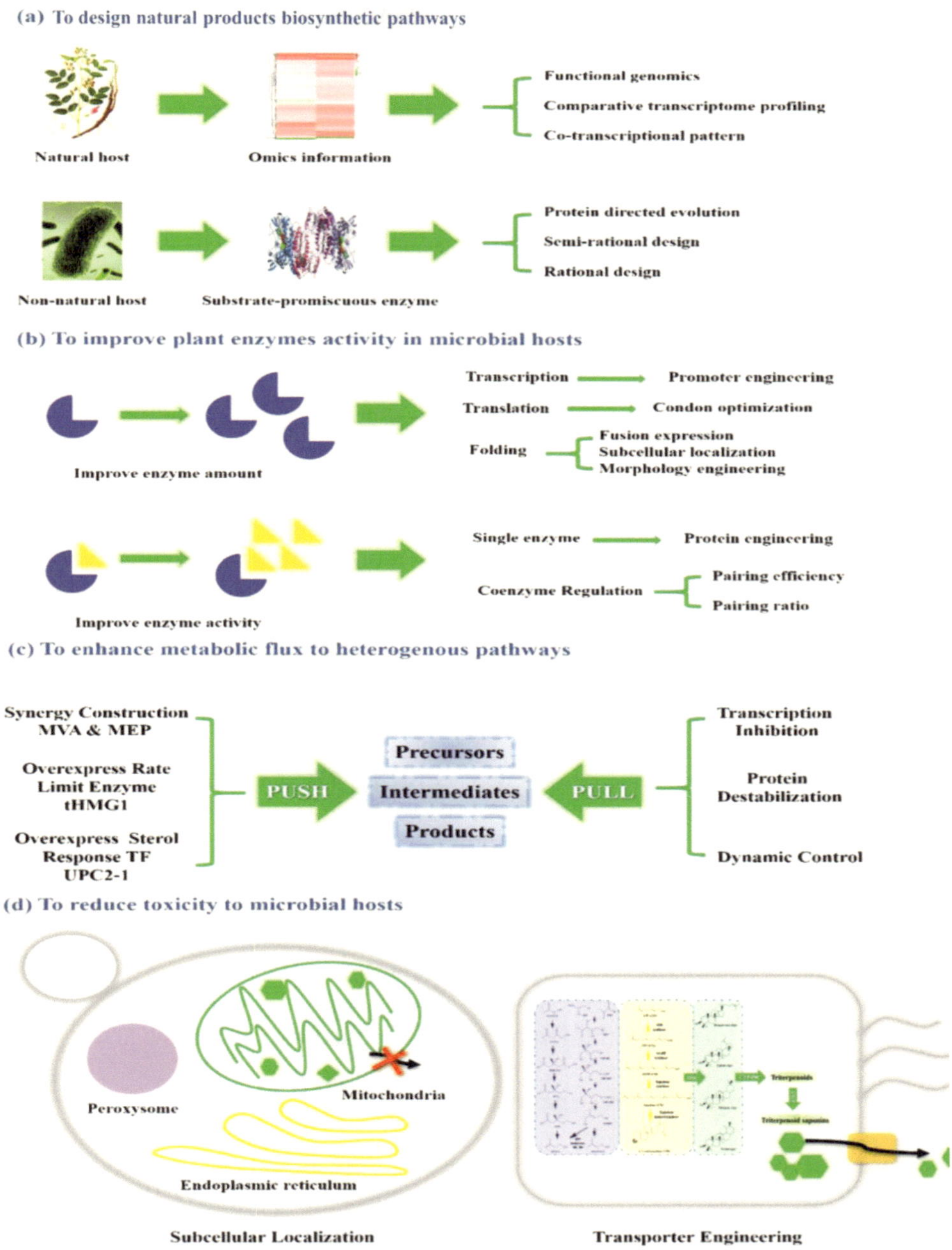

Figure 3.
Scheme for strategies used to advance biosynthesis of triterpenoid saponins in microbial hosts. (a) Strategies to design triterpenoid saponins biosynthetic pathways; (b) Strategies to improve plant enzyme activity in microbial hosts; (c) Strategies to enhance metabolic flux in microbial hosts; (d) Strategies to reduce toxicity to the hosts.

through comparing the transcriptome data between high- and low-producing varieties, the genes including bAS1, CYP716A79 and CYP716A78 that involved in quinoa saponins biosynthesis were targeted from *Chenopodium quinoa*. The predicted genes were then functionally identified by expressing in yeast [32]. By comparing the transcriptome data between ethyl alcohol and methyl jasmonate elicited conditions, key genes involved in maesasaponins biosynthesis including bAS, CYP716A75 and CYP87D16 from *Maesa lanceolate* were targeted and were subsequently identified by expressing in yeast host [33]. Depending on the comparison of the transcriptome data between varieties with different phenotype, key genes involved in target compound biosynthetic pathways can be predicted, and be further identified by functionally expressed in yeast. Generally, the expression patterns of genes involved in the same biological process are strongly correlated. Thus, genes co-expression analysis was applied to predict the functions of unidentified genes. Based on this strategy, CYP716A12, CYP93E2, CYP72A61v2 and CYP72A68v2 from *M. truncatula* have been functionally identified [34].

Besides mining enzymes from native host, the application of the substrate-promiscuous enzymes turned out to be an alternative approach to reconstruct the target compounds biosynthetic pathways. For instance, the nonnative substrate-promiscuous glycosyltransferase Bs-YjiC from *B. subtilis* 168 was used for the synthesis of ginsenoside Rh1 and some unnatural ginsenosides in *S. cerevisiae* [35]. Other substrate-promiscuous enzymes like UDP-glycosyltransferase UGT109A1, was also used to produce the unnatural ginsenosides 3β, 12β-Di-O-Glc-PPD, 3β,12β-Di-O-Glc-PPT, 3β,20S-Di-O-Glc-DM, and 3β-O-Glc-DM.

The low final concentration of the synthesized compounds is always caused by the poor enzyme activity on the unnatural substrate. Protein evaluation, which could improve the catalytic characteristic involving "substrate specificity" of the substrate-promiscuous enzymes has been developed for the specific decoration of natural and unnatural substrates. One example is the engineering of the substrate-promiscuous UDP-glucose sterol glucosyltransferase UGT51 from *S. cerevisiae*. UGT51 can glycosylate a series of structural analogues, including pregnenolone, cholesterol, ergosterol, sitosterol, diosgenin, estradiol, PPD and PPT. Because of the wide substrate spectrum, UGT51 has been applied for the biosynthesis of ginsenosides Rh2 with the co-expression of PgDS, CYP716A47 and AtCPR1 in *S. cerevisiae*. However, only trace amount of Rh2 was synthesized. To improve the enzyme activity, a semi-rational design strategy was developed based on the crystal structure of UGT51 (PDB code: 5gl5). The best UGT51 mutant gained an 1800-fold higher catalytic efficiency (kcat/Km) in converting PPD to ginsenoside Rh2 in vitro and the Rh2 production reached up to 300 mg/L in vivo [35]. Using non-native promiscuous enzymes to reconstruct the natural products biosynthetic pathways is an efficient strategy to achieve the heterogeneous synthesis of triterpenoid saponins in yeast, especially for that without integrated illuminated pathways.

4.2 Strategies to improve plant enzyme activity

Plant CYP450s are indispensable enzymes for the C–H bounds oxidation of triterpenoid skeletons. However, heterogeneous expression of plant CYP450s in yeasts hosts usually exists problems as low expression level, poor catalytic efficiency or even incorrect folding structure. Plant CYP450s involved in triterpenoids synthesis are membrane-bound oxidase enzymes, which anchor in the endoplasmic reticulum (ER) of plants cells and requires electrons transferred by CYP450 reductase. Although CYP450 is essential for the hydroxylation of C–H bounds and can further oxidize the alcohol products to aldehyde and acid, it always shows poor activity on such substrates. As a result, it is challenging to establish high-yield triterpenoid saponins in yeast cell factories, and improving the plant CYP450s is essential to improve the situation. Currently, many strategies have been developed to improve the expression level and regulate the pairing efficiency of CPRs to plant CYP450s in microbial hosts.

Codon optimization and application of a strong promoter are the most common strategies to improve enzyme expression level in heterologous hosts and it is also effectively used to improve plant CYP450s expression level in microbial hosts [36]. Chimeric protein has been used to correct the folding of plant CYP450s in microbial hosts. As plant CYP450s are anchored in ER membrane, the activity can be improved by replacing the native N-terminal sequence with ER-membrane bound proteins of yeast to facilitate correctly folding and anchoring. Protein directed evolution was also applied to enhance the activity of plant enzymes. In consideration of that the enlargement of ER would provide more room for the ER-located CYP450s and CPRs leading to higher protein abundance, a novel ER morphology engineering strategy is developed. Through the deletion of PAH1 gene encoding phosphatidic acid phosphatase, the ER membranes of *S. cerevisiae* was tremendously expanded, which accelerated the expression of CYP450s including CYP716A12, CYP72A67 and CYP72A68, and ultimately leading to increased production of triterpenoid and triterpenoid saponins. Approaches like codon optimization, Chimeric protein, protein directed evolution and ER enlargement have been used to improve CYP450s expression level in heterologous hosts.

The pairing efficiency of CYP450s and CPRs plays an important role for the catalytic activity of CYP450s. Mining novel CPRs is a straightforward way to improve the CYP450 activities as different CPRs has different pairing efficiency with CYP450s. For example, the CPR from *M. truncatula* was proved to be the most efficient one pairing with CYP716A12 among all the tested CPRs from *G. uralensis*, *Lotus japonicus* and *A. thaliana*, and boosted OA biosynthesis in yeast [15]. Moreover, the co-expression of CYP72A63 and/or uni25647 with GuCPR1 from *G. uralensis* showed higher activities than the co-expression with other CPRs from *M. truncatula*, *A. thaliana*, or *L. japonicus*. The using of GuCPR1 resulted in boosted GA production in yeast [14]. Besides the using different CPRs, ratios between CYP450 and CPR also contribute to the CYP450 activities. Fine-tuning the ratios between CYP450 and CPR is an important strategy to improve their pairing efficiency. For example, with the best ratio of 5:9 between CYP716Y1 and CPR1 from *A. thaliana*, the 16-α-hydroxy amyrin production was significantly increased [30]. These results indicate that improving the pairing efficiency by efficient CPRs and proper pairing ratio between CYP450 and CPR can improve the targeted compound production in yeast.

4.3 Strategies to enhance metabolic flux

The plant natural products biosynthetic pathways always include multiple steps. When introduced in yeast, the heterogeneous pathways would intensively interact with the native metabolic network, by means of competing substrates and co-factors as well as metabolites reverse influence. The disturbance will restrict the targeted compound production. Therefore, balancing metabolic flux distribution between heterologous pathways and native metabolic networks plays an important role in promoting the production of targeted compound.

Enhancing the precursors supplement to the targeted pathway is a straightforward strategy to enhance natural products production. As demonstrated, the five-carbon building blocks IPP and DMAPP are naturally synthesized through either eukaryotic MVA or prokaryotic MEP pathway in microorganisms. The combination of MVA and MEP pathways in one host could take advantages of both pathways and lead to more efficient precursor supplement for terpenoids. Through introducing a heterogeneous MVA pathway, 27.0 g/L amorphadiene was achieved in *E. coli*. Besides, the production of other terpenoids such as valerenadiene (62.0 mg/L), isoprene (24.0 g/L), and lycopene (47.0 mg/L) were also successfully increased by the synergy of the MEP and the MVA pathway in *E. coli*. In view of the availability of this strategy, the combination of MVA and MEP pathway have been developed in yeast. In addition to the cooperation of the MEP and the MVA pathways, taking full advantage of precursors synthesized in different organelles was helpful to boost the terpenoids producing. By improving the utilization of acetyl-CoA through the simultaneously introducing dual MVA pathways located in cytoplasmic and mitochondrial of yeast, 2.5 mg/L isoprene was obtained [37]. Moreover, HMG-CoA reductase catalyzing the conversion of HMG-CoA to mevalonate is a rate-limiting factor of MVA pathway. The HMG-CoA reductase is feedback regulated due to its N-term transmembrane sequence, so the truncated version (N-term truncated) of HMG-CoA reductase (tHMG1) is intensively used to strengthen the precursor supplement. Globe transcriptional regulation by overexpressing UPC2-1, which is a global sterol regulatory element to induce sterol biosynthetic genes expression, is another effective method to improve the MVA flux globally [38].

Decreasing the metabolic flux of competing pathways is efficient to strengthen the flux to targeted pathway. However, in most cases, directly deletion of the enzymes involved in the competing could lead to lethality, for many of the genes are essential to the hosts. Therefore, decrease the metabolic flux to the competing pathways by down-regulation of key enzymes is a proper approach to strengthen the final production. Generally, the cellular protein concentration is regulated by transcription, RNA degradation, translation and protein degradation. The application of weaker promoters is the most commonly used strategy to down-regulate the transcriptional level of key genes. To decrease the sterol synthesis and redirect the metabolic flux to the β-amyrin synthesis pathway in yeast. ERG7 (lanosterol synthase gene) promoter was replaced by a methionine repressible promoter (PMET3). Moreover, in order to improve the α-santalene accumulation in yeast, the native promoter of ERG9 (squalene synthase gene) was replaced by PCRT3, the copper repressible promoter and PHXT1, a low concentration glucose repressible promoter which resulted in decreased metabolic flux to ergosterol synthesis and increased α-santalene production [39]. Recently, dynamic protein degradation was developed to weaken the competing pathways. Depending on the ER-associated protein degradation system, the cytosolic proteins can be degraded when attached by a PEST sequence. As a result, the strategy of using the G1 cyclin PEST sequence as a degradation degron to label the cytosolic term of squalene synthase was developed for the production of trans-nerolidol. Once labeled by degron, the squalene synthase will be degraded dynamically, resulting in enhanced sesquiterpene trans-nerolidol production. By the similar strategy, farnesyl pyrophosphate synthetase was labeled by a designed N-terminal degron on the N-terminus, which increased the titer of monoterpene linalool [40].

4.4 Strategies to reduce toxicity to the hosts

Natural products always exhibit cytotoxicity to the microbial hosts, leading to decreased cell growth and finally impair the production. In order to solve these problems, various strategies were developed including two-stage fermentation, pathway compartmentalization and transporters mediated compound secretion. In order to alleviate the negative influences on cell growth, the fermentation course is divided into two stages. In first fermentation stage, heterogeneous pathway keep silence and cells grow fast with precursor accumulated, while in the second stage, target pathway would be induced to produce the target compounds [41]. In addition to the traditional two-stage fermentation, the organelles including mitochondria, peroxisome and vacuole were also used to compartmentalize the heterogeneous pathways. Because the integrated membrane structure, these organelles are relatively independent from the cytoplasm, which could prevent the toxic precursors and products from distributing in cytoplasm to disrupt cell growth. Furthermore, subcellular compartmentalization of target biosynthetic pathways can concentrate the substrates, intermediates and enzymes in a more narrow space, which can improve the reaction efficiency of enzymes. Through locating the amorpha-4,11-diene biosynthetic pathways in the mitochondria of yeast, the amorpha-4,11-diene production increased by 63% compared with locating in the cytosol. By this strategy, the precursor FPP was restricted in mitochondria by the membrane structure, which reduced the loss of FPP. Using similar strategy, the valencene biosynthetic pathway was reconstructed into the mitochondria of yeast resulting in eight-fold increase of valencene production. Besides the mitochondria, peroxisome was also used to compartmentalize the heterogeneous pathways, by introducing the lycopene synthesis pathway in peroxisome, lycopene production was improved up to 73.9 mg/L in Pichia pastoris [42]. Therefore, subcellular compartmentalization was a pioneering strategy to reduce products cytotoxicity to the microbial hosts.

Another strategy to reduce the inner cytotoxicity of natural products is to secrete these compounds outside the cell automatically. To achieve this goal, transporters were taken into account, for their significant contribution of transporting the products to the extracellular space. Due to the rarity of transporters that possess the ability to transport the complex natural products, transporter engineering has been developed to improve the situation. For example, through protein engineering, one variant of AcrB from AcrAB-TolC efflux pump can effectively improve the α-pinene efflux out of the *E. coli* cell. However, because of unclear of the transport mechanisms and lacking of crystal structures, the application of transporters in natural products is still limited.

In this chapter, the biosynthetic pathways of natural products and their reconstruction in yeast cell factories were systematically summarized. The strategies developed to increase natural products productivity in yeast were also discussed including protein engineering, metabolic engineering, subcellular localization and fermentation control. With these endeavors, the engineered strains can produce these compounds in different levels. These achievements indicate yeast a promising chassis for the heterogeneous biosynthesis of natural products.

Acknowledgements

The authors kindly acknowledge financial support from the National Science Fund for Distinguished Young Scholars (NO. 21425624) and the National Natural Science Foundation of China (NO. 21506011, NO. 21476026).

Author details

Wentao Sun, Yu-jia Zhao and Chun Li*
Department of Biochemical Engineering, School of Chemistry and Chemical Engineering, Institute for Synthetic Biosystem, Beijing Institute of Technology, Beijing, China

*Address all correspondence to: lichun@bit.edu.cn

References

[1] Thimmappa R, Geisler K, Louveau T, et al. Triterpene biosynthesis in plants. Annual Review of Plant Biology. 2014;**65**:225-257. DOI: 10.1146/annurev-arplant-050312-120229

[2] Scognamiglio M, D'Abrosca B, Fiumano V, et al. Oleanane saponins from *Bellis sylvestris* Cyr. and evaluation of their phytotoxicity on Aegilops geniculata Roth. Phytochemistry. 2012;**84**(12):125-134

[3] Zhao Y, Lv B, Feng X, et al. Perspective on biotransformation and de novo biosynthesis of licorice constituents. Journal of Agricultural and Food Chemistry. 2017;**65**(51): 11147-11156. DOI: 10.1021/acs.jafc.7b04470

[4] Wang L, Weller CL. Recent advances in extraction of nutraceuticals from plants. Trends in Food Science & Technology. 2006;**17**(6):300-312

[5] Pablo P, Catalina P, Manuel RC. New insights into plant isoprenoid metabolism. Molecular Plant. 2012;**5**(5):964-967

[6] Zheyong X, Lixin D, Dan L, et al. Divergent evolution of oxidosqualene cyclases in plants. New Phytologist. 2012;**193**(4):1022-1038

[7] Aragão GF, Carneiro LMV, Júnior APF, et al. Antiplatelet activity of α.- and β.-Amyrin, isomeric mixture from Protium heptaphyllum. Pharmaceutical Biology. 2007;**45**(5):343-349

[8] Augustin JM, Kuzina V, Andersen SB, et al. Molecular activities, biosynthesis and evolution of triterpenoid saponins. Phytochemistry. 2011;**72**(6):435-457. DOI: 10.1016/j.phytochem.2011.01.015

[9] Loew GH, Harris DL. Role of the heme active site and protein environment in structure, spectra, and function of the cytochrome p450s. Chemical Reviews. 2010;**31**(16):407-420

[10] Yasumoto S, Fukushima EO, Seki H, et al. Novel triterpene oxidizing activity of *Arabidopsis thaliana* CYP716A subfamily enzymes. FEBS Letters. 2016;**590**(4):533-540. DOI: 10.1002/1873-3468.12074

[11] Zhang R, Li C, Wang J, et al. Microbial production of small medicinal molecules and biologics: From nature to synthetic pathways. Biotechnology Advances. 2018;**36**(8):2219-2231. DOI: 10.1016/j.biotechadv.2018.10.009

[12] Li Y, Li S, Thodey K, et al. Complete biosynthesis of noscapine and halogenated alkaloids in yeast. Proceedings of the National Academy of Sciences of the United States of America. 2018:**115**(17):3922-3931

[13] Zhang G, Cao Q, Liu J, et al. Refactoring β-amyrin synthesis in *Saccharomyces cerevisiae*. AICHE Journal. 2015;**61**(10):3172-3179. DOI: 10.1002/aic.14950

[14] Zhu M, Wang C, Sun W, et al. Boosting 11-oxo-beta-amyrin and glycyrrhetinic acid synthesis in *Saccharomyces cerevisiae* via pairing novel oxidation and reduction system from legume plants. Metabolic Engineering. 2018;**45**:43-50. DOI: 10.1016/j.ymben.2017.11.009

[15] Zhao Y, Fan J, Wang C, et al. Enhancing oleanolic acid production in engineered *Saccharomyces cerevisiae*. Bioresource Technology. 2018;**257**:339-343. DOI: 10.1016/j.biortech.2018.02.096

[16] Yu Y, Chang P, Yu H, et al. Productive Amyrin Synthases for efficient alpha-amyrin synthesis in engineered *Saccharomyces cerevisiae*. ACS Synthetic Biology. 2018;**7**(10):2391-2402. DOI: 10.1021/acssynbio.8b00176

[17] Liu X, Zhang L, Feng X, et al. Biosynthesis of glycyrrhetinic acid-3-O-monoglucose using glycosyltransferase UGT73C11 from *Barbarea vulgaris*. Industrial & Engineering Chemistry Research. 2017;**56**(51):14949-14958. DOI: 10.1021/acs.iecr.7b03391

[18] Endale M, Lee WM, Kamruzzaman SM, et al. Ginsenoside-Rp1 inhibits platelet activation and thrombus formation via impaired glycoprotein VI signalling pathway, tyrosine phosphorylation and MAPK activation. British Journal of Pharmacology. 2012;**167**(1):109-127

[19] Han JY, Kim HJ, Kwon YS, et al. The Cyt P450 enzyme CYP716A47 catalyzes the formation of protopanaxadiol from dammarenediol-II during ginsenoside biosynthesis in *Panax ginseng*. Plant & Cell Physiology. 2011;**52**(12):2062-2073. DOI: 10.1093/pcp/pcr150

[20] Han JY, Kim MJ, Ban YW, et al. The involvement of β-amyrin 28-oxidase (CYP716A52v2) in oleanane-type ginsenoside biosynthesis in *Panax ginseng*. Plant & Cell Physiology. 2013;**54**(12):2034-2046

[21] Dai Z, Liu Y, Zhang X, et al. Metabolic engineering of *Saccharomyces cerevisiae* for production of ginsenosides. Metabolic Engineering. 2013;**20**(5):146-156

[22] Suk-Chae J, Woohyun K, Sung Chul P, et al. Two ginseng UDP-glycosyltransferases synthesize ginsenoside Rg3 and Rd. Plant & Cell Physiology. 2014;**55**(12):2177

[23] Wei W, Wang P, Wei Y, et al. Characterizations of *Panax ginseng* UDP-glycosyltransferases catalyzing protopanaxatriol and biosyntheses of bioactive ginsenosides F1 and Rh1 in metabolically engineered yeasts. Molecular Plant. 2015;**8**(9):1412-1424

[24] Quan LH, Min JW, Yang DU, et al. Enzymatic biotransformation of ginsenoside Rb1 to 20()-Rg3 by recombinant β-glucosidase from Microbacterium esteraromaticum. Applied Microbiology and Biotechnology. 2012;**94**(2):377-384

[25] Chen J, Wu H, Wang Q, et al. Ginsenoside metabolite compound K alleviates adjuvant-induced arthritis by suppressing T cell activation. Inflammation. 2014;**37**(5):1608-1615

[26] Xing Y, Yun F, Wei W, et al. Production of bioactive ginsenoside compound K in metabolically engineered yeast. Cell Research. 2014;**24**(6):770-773

[27] Liang H, Hu Z, Zhang T, et al. Production of a bioactive unnatural ginsenoside by metabolically engineered yeasts based on a new UDP-glycosyltransferase from *Bacillus subtilis*. Metabolic Engineering. 2017;**44**:60

[28] Itkin M, Davidovich-Rikanati R, Cohen S, et al. The biosynthetic pathway of the nonsugar, high-intensity sweetener mogroside V from Siraitia grosvenorii. Proceedings of the National Academy of Sciences of the United States of America. 2016;**113**(47):E7619

[29] Aoyagi H, Kobayashi Y, Yamada K, et al. Efficient production of saikosaponins in *Bupleurum falcatum* root fragments combined with signal transducers. Applied Microbiology and Biotechnology. 2001;**57**(4):482-488

[30] Tessa M, Jacob P, Lorena A, et al. Combinatorial biosynthesis of sapogenins and saponins in *Saccharomyces cerevisiae* using a C-16α hydroxylase from *Bupleurum falcatum*. Proceedings of the National Academy of Sciences of the United States of America. 2014;**111**(4):1634-1639

[31] Ma T, Shi B, Ye Z, et al. Lipid engineering combined with systematic metabolic engineering of *Saccharomyces*

cerevisiae for high-yield production of lycopene. Metabolic Engineering. 2019;**52**:134-142. DOI: 10.1016/j.ymben.2018.11.009

[32] Fiallos-Jurado J, Pollier J, Moses T, et al. Saponin determination, expression analysis and functional characterization of saponin biosynthetic genes in *Chenopodium quinoa* leaves. Plant Science. 2016;**250**:188-197

[33] Moses T, Pollier J, Faizal A, et al. Unraveling the triterpenoid saponin biosynthesis of the African shrub *Maesa lanceolata*. Molecular Plant. 2015;**8**(1):122-135. DOI: 10.1016/j.molp.2014.11.004

[34] Fukushima EO, Seki H, Sawai S, et al. Combinatorial biosynthesis of legume natural and rare triterpenoids in engineered yeast. Plant & Cell Physiology. 2013;**54**(5):740-749. DOI: 10.1093/pcp/pct015

[35] Dai L, Li J, Yang J, et al. Use of a promiscuous glycosyltransferase from *Bacillus subtilis* 168 for the enzymatic synthesis of novel protopanaxatriol-type ginsenosides. Journal of Agricultural and Food Chemistry. 2018;**66**(4):943-949

[36] Nybo SE, Saunders J, Mccormick SP. Metabolic engineering of *Escherichia coli* for production of valerenadiene. Journal of Biotechnology. 2017;**262**:60-66

[37] Lv X, Wang F, Zhou P, et al. Dual regulation of cytoplasmic and mitochondrial acetyl-CoA utilization for improved isoprene production in *Saccharomyces cerevisiae*. Nature Communications. 2016;**7**:12851. DOI: 10.1038/ncomms12851

[38] Zhubo D, Yi L, Luqi H, et al. Production of miltiradiene by metabolically engineered *Saccharomyces cerevisiae*. Biotechnology and Bioengineering. 2012;**109**(11):2845-2853

[39] Koch B, Schacher G, Inc HLR. Dynamic control of gene expression in *Saccharomyces cerevisiae* engineered for the production of plant sesquitepene α-santalene in a fed-batch mode. Metabolic Engineering. 2012;**14**(2):91-103

[40] Peng B, Nielsen LK, Kampranis SC, et al. Engineered protein degradation of farnesyl pyrophosphate synthase is an effective regulatory mechanism to increase monoterpene production in *Saccharomyces cerevisiae*. Metabolic Engineering. 2018;**47**:83-93

[41] Pingping Z, Lidan Y, Wenping X, et al. Highly efficient biosynthesis of astaxanthin in *Saccharomyces cerevisiae* by integration and tuning of algal crtZ and bkt. Applied Microbiology and Biotechnology. 2015;**99**(20):8419-8428

[42] Bhataya A, Schmidt-Dannert C, Lee PC. Metabolic engineering of Pichia pastoris X-33 for lycopene production. Process Biochemistry. 2009;**44**(10):1095-1102